MYOCARDIAL INFARCTION IN WOMEN

MYOCARDIAL INFARCTION IN WOMEN

Edited by

Michael F. Oliver
Anders Vedin
Claes Wilhelmsson

Cardiovascular Research Unit, University of Edinburgh, UK, and Section of Preventive Cardiology, Östra Hospital, Göteborg, Sweden

CHURCHILL LIVINGSTONE
EDINBURGH LONDON MELBOURNE AND NEW YORK 1986

CHURCHILL LIVINGSTONE
Medical Division of Longman Group UK Limited

Distributed in the United States of America by
Churchill Livingstone Inc., 1560 Broadway, New
York, N.Y. 10036, and by associated companies,
branches and representatives throughout the world.

First published 1986

ISBN 0 443 03743 4

British Library Cataloguing in Publication Data
Myocardial infarction in women.
    1. Heart—Infarction   2. Women—Diseases
    I. Oliver, Michael F.   II. Vedin, Anders
    III. Wilhelmsson, Claes
    616.1'237'0088042   RC685.16

Library of Congress Cataloging in Publication Data
Myocardial infarction in women
    Includes index
    1. Heart—infarction.   2. Women—diseases.
    I. Oliver, M. F. (Michael Francis)   II. Vedin, Anders.
    III. Wilhelmsson, Claes [DNLM: 1. Myocardial
    Infarction. WG 300 M99736]
    RC685.16M8974   1986   616.1'237'088042   86-13723

Printed at The Bath Press, Avon

Preface

The relative infrequency of myocardial infarction among women has intrigued physicians and scientists for many years. In 1978 a meeting was held in Edinburgh, Scotland, in order to establish 'the state of the art'. Since then, several studies have been reported and many important facts have been presented. Therefore we felt that it was timely to take the initiative once again to gather active scientists in the field in an effort to establish the current level of our knowledge and provide an in-depth analysis of the sex differences regarding ischaemic heart disease.

Only established workers in the area were invited. Thus, this book may serve as a platform of reference and be useful also to those who want an updated account of present affairs.

Hässle/Astra Cardiovascular have very generously provided the necessary financial support for this venture, not only in organising the meeting but also in undertaking editorial responsibilities and coordination of the publication.

M.F.O.
A.V.
C.W.

1986

v

Contributors

J.-L. Beaumont
Unité de Recherches sur l'Athérosclérose, INSERM U 32, Hôpital Henri-Mondor, Créteil, France

V. Beaumont
Unité de Recherches sur l'Athérosclérose, INSERM U 32, Hôpital Henri-Mondor, Créteil, France

C. Bengtsson
Department of Medicine II, Sahlgrenska Hospital, University of Göteborg, Göteborg, Sweden

H.J. Engel
Division of Cardiology, Zentralkrankenhaus 'Links der Weser', Bremen, FRG

F.H. Epstein
Institut für Sozial- und Präventivmedizin, Universität Zürich, Zürich Switzerland

S.G. Haynes
Department of Epidemiology, University of North Carolina, Chapel Hill, NC, USA

S. Johansson
Section of Preventive Cardiology, Department of Medicine, Östra Hospital, Göteborg, Sweden

E.A. Nikkilä
Third Department of Medicine, University of Helsinki Hospital, Helsinki, Finland

M.F. Oliver
Cardiovascular Research Unit, University of Edinburgh, Edinburgh, UK

A. Reunanen
Research Institute for Social Security, the Social Insurance Institution, Helsinki, Finland

B.M. Rifkind
Lipid Metabolism Atherogenesis Branch, National Institutes of Health, Bethesda, MD, USA

A.M. Rissanen
Department of Public Health, University of Tampere and Third Department of Medicine, University of Helsinki, Helsinki, Finland

L. Rosenberg
Drug Epidemiology Unit, School of Public Health, Boston University School of Medicine, Brookline, MA, USA

S. Shapiro
Drug Epidemiology Unit, School of Public Health, Boston University School of Medicine, Brookline, MA, USA

J. Slack
Clinical Genetics Department, Royal Free Hospital, London, UK

N.H. Sternby
University Department of Pathology, General Hospital, Malmö, Sweden

A. Vedin
Section of Preventive Cardiology, Department of Medicine, Östra Hospital, Göteborg, Sweden

R.J. Weir
Division of Medicine and MRC Blood Pressure Unit, Western Infirmary, Glasgow, UK

C. Wilhelmsson
Section of Preventive Cardiology, Department of Medicine, Östra Hospital, Göteborg, Sweden

V. Wynn
The Alexander Simpson Laboratory for Metabolic Research, St. Mary's Hospital Medical School, University of London, London, UK

Contents

1. Mortality, time trends and sex differences in coronary heart disease

F.H. Epstein

MORTALITY AND TIME TRENDS

For a good many years it has been known that coronary heart disease (CHD) is more common in men than women and that the difference varies from country to country. In general, as heart disease mortality rises in men, the male/female ratio increases (Table 1.1). The data shown[1] are averages for the years 1975–78 and 'heart

Table 1.1 Male/female ratios of death rates for heart disease*, ages 45–64, in the years 1975–78 and average percent change † between 1950 and 1978

Country	Sex ratio 1975–78	Average change (%)
Finland	5.00	+ 14.2
Norway	4.76	+ 15.4
Sweden	4.40	+ 18.4
Netherlands	4.29	+ 17.1
Canada	3.74	+ 8.9
Denmark	3.73	+ 10.8
England and Wales	3.66	+ 7.0
France	3.61	+ 12.5
Switzerland	3.61	+ 10.0
FRG	3.33	+ 12.4
USA	3.47	+ 4.6
Czechoslovakia	3.36	+ 9.8
Belgium	3.30	+ 12.9
Austria	3.27	+ 6.0
Poland	3.17	+ 11.9
New Zealand	3.16	+ 5.7
Australia	3.15	+ 4.0
Ireland	3.09	+ 16.1
Northern Ireland	3.08	+ 10.5
Scotland	3.05	+ 5.2
Italy	2.88	+ 14.2
Spain	2.84	+ 12.0
Portugal	2.42	+ 8.4
Israel	2.14	+ 0.0
Japan	2.09	+ 8.6
Yugoslavia	1.87	+ 13.8

* Age-adjusted
† Average change every 5 years based on log linear slope

1

disease' is defined as 'non-rheumatic and hypertensive heart disease' in order to analyse 30 year time trends as will be done later, because over the years the category 'ischaemic heart disease' has changed its definition in the International Classification of Causes of Death. The rates, as in all subsequent analyses, are age-standardised over the range 45–64 years. There is, indeed, an overall correlation. At the same time, the scatter is rather large so that the ratio in countries like the Netherlands or Sweden is considerably higher than in the Federal Republic of Germany, Belgium, Austria and Poland which have similar death rates in men. While such ratios are sensitive to small differences in rates in either direction, the differences between the countries mentioned are due to slightly lower rates among women in the Netherlands and Sweden since the rates for men are similar. It is not immediately apparent why more women should die of heart disease relative to men in England and Wales than in the Irish Republic. It is all very well to ask questions but there is little point in it unless there is a reasonable chance that they can be answered. International mortality data have been useful points of departure for further research in the past and the same may be hoped from the kind of analyses presented here.

Moving on to trends over time (Fig. 1.1), mortality from heart disease in the same 26 countries has been arranged in order of descending rates among men in 1950–54 for five further time periods. The detailed data are being published.[1] The contour lines demarcating the range between the highest and lowest rate from country to country are shown here. A striking pattern emerges. Geographical differences are much more marked for men than women, making it apparent why the sex ratio is so

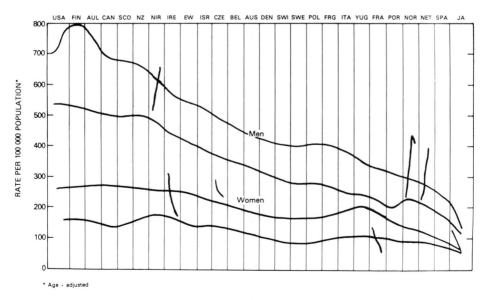

Fig. 1.1 Death rates for heart disease in men and women aged 45–64; 26 countries, 1950–78. The upper and lower lines for each sex demarcate the range in which death rates moved up or down in six time periods between 1950 and 1978. The trend lines for Northern Ireland (NIR), Ireland (IRE), Czechoslovakia (CZE), France (FRA), Norway (NOR) and the Netherlands (NET) fell outside the range and were drawn individually for each of these countries in the appropriate sex group.

much lower in some countries than others. There is some tendency for time trends in men to decrease in countries where they were originally high and to rise where they were low, with France and Japan being exceptions.[1] In women, the trend is invariably and continuously downwards since 1950.[1] It is worthy of note that countries maintained their relative positions, the changes over time having been insufficient to alter the overall pattern.

When *total* death rates among men are again arranged in order of descending heart disease rates, geographical variation is somewhat less marked and the pattern is more ragged.[1] Eight countries with low mortalities in men stand out: Israel, Denmark, Switzerland, Sweden, Norway, the Netherlands, Spain and Japan (after a spectacular drop). In the first four countries, the total mortality is lower than might be expected in terms of heart disease. In women, the trend for total mortality is again inexorably downwards.[1]

It was of interest to see whether countries with a high sex ratio at the present time had a greater average change in the sex ratio since 1950 (Table 1.1). It is true that a cluster of four countries with the highest sex ratio were in the highest range of change. Even so, with sex ratios between 3:1 and 4:1 which encompass the majority of countries, almost any degree of change can be found. Perhaps, it is not surprising to get a vague answer to a vague question.

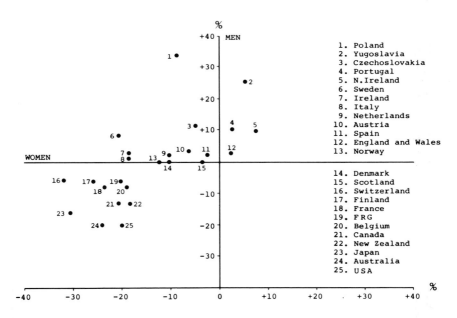

Fig. 1.2 Percent change in death rates for heart disease by sex and country, ages 45–64, 1965/69 to 1975/78.

At the World Heart Congress in 1966, data were shown which suggested that countries in which CHD mortality rose most in the 1950s and early 1960s among men also showed the least decline in women.[2] The inference was drawn that a detrimental environment affects the most susceptible sex preferentially and puts a

3

brake on the natural downwards course seen in women who are relatively resistent to the disease. This relationship still seems to hold on comparing percentage changes in death rates from 'heart disease', as defined here, in men and women between the late 1960s and the late 70s (Fig. 1.2). Again there is a remarkable parallel so far as countries which show greater rises or falls in men also tend to show greater respective rises or falls in women. Hence, even though secular trends are divergent in the two sexes in many countries, environmental influences, favourable or detrimental, still affect men and women in the same direction. This is a powerful argument in support of the view that, in spite of all the sex differences in susceptibility toward CHD and atherosclerosis, preventive measures are likely to be similarly effective in men and women.

DISCUSSION

It must be emphasised that this general view, ending with the year 1978, has not addressed the question whether or to what extent—and where—the downward trends for women may have recently flattened out or even been reversed, most particularly in the younger age groups. Such data, relating particularly to the use of contraceptives and changing smoking habits among women, are much needed. Another need is to analyse the trends by social class which is unfortunately possible only in Britain, thanks to the foresight of the Registrar-General in providing this information. The newly developing community projects with their registers may yield some such data within the limitations of numbers.

The data which have been presented are clearly required as background for a discussion of CHD in women. While a picture needs a frame, it is the picture which really matters. Has anything been learnt? Many questions remain open. It is still largely unknown why CHD mortality is lower in women. Saying that women develop coronary atherosclerosis more slowly than men begs the question of why this should be so. Besides, it is possible if not likely that some of the protection is related to myocardial factors, apart from the amount of atherosclerosis and these again may be related in part to the reasons for geographical and time-trend differences. In any case, it would seem that mortality in men is a sensitive indicator for environmental determinants of the disease and that women respond to them in a similar way but—on account of protective factors—on a lower absolute level of disease incidence.

For further progress there is every reason to keep the type of mortality surveillance presented there up to date in order to discern any change in pattern which might be a sentinel for the emergence of new influences or the continuing activity of presently operative environmental and risk factors. From the point of view of research, it would seem equally or even more important to take the data already at hand and look for any incongruities in the findings between women and men, analysing in detail and in comparable fashion the situation in two or more countries and trying to find an explanation. Here are some examples:

1. At similar current male rates, the sex ratio is much higher in Norway than Belgium or in Finland than Scotland.

2. In Ireland, female rates declined steeply while the rate in men climbed

moderately; in Norway and the Netherlands, rates in women diminished very little while there was a steep rise in the rates for men.

3. In the two most recent time periods analysed, the female rate decreased to the same extent in Sweden and the Federal Republic of Germany or Belgium, but in Sweden the male rate went up and in the other two countries down.

In assessing the situation and selecting the countries that tell us most, it must be kept in mind that a small absolute change in a country with initially low mortality will express itself as a rather large percentage change, as in Japan, or, to a lesser degree, in Sweden. Conversely, a large absolute change in a country with initially high mortality may present as a relatively small percentage change. Hence, presenting the data both in absolute and percentage terms rather than in relative terms only, as was largely done up to now, is important.

SUMMARY

Mortality trends from 'heart disease' (non-rheumatic heart disease and hypertension) between the years 1950 and 1978 in 26 countries have been described. Geographical variation is much more pronounced in men than in women, rates have decreased uniformly in women but not in men, and changes in mortality during the 28 year period have not altered the relative position of countries along the scale from high to low death rates. The male/female mortality ratios vary widely from country to country but bear little relation to secular changes in this ratio. It is important to continue monitoring the heart disease mortality trends in the two sexes in the years to come, with particular attention to countries where particular features of the pattern of change in women and men might help to discover the factors responsible for differential secular trends.

REFERENCES

[1] Thom T, Epstein F H, Feldman J, Leaverton P E. Trends in total mortality and mortality from heart disease in 26 countries from 1950–78. Int J Epidemiol 1985; 14: 510–520.
[2] Epstein F H. Coronary heart disease at younger ages. Symposia du Ve Congres Mondial de Cardiologie. Acta Cardiol (Brux) 1968: 345–53.

Discussion on Chapter 1

Oliver
One of the most striking aspects of the secular changes in coronary disease and total mortality is the consistent downward trends in women which occurred as early as between 1950 and 1960 and well ahead of any of the major preventive campaigns and in countries where preventive campaigns are not very active even now.

Epstein
The change has been upward or downward in men but consistently downward in women, which is still a mystery. Some of the changes in the last 10 years, particularly the decline in the United States, are reasonably specific, relating to nutrition, blood pressure control and smoking. Beyond this, better social conditions make for better health.

Oliver
My question was specifically related to the downward trends in women that took place between 1950 and 1960. The changes that may have occurred in men during the last 10 years are a different issue. Is there any evidence that there was more improvement in medical care and social conditions for women than for men 25 years ago?

Haynes
Medical care use has always been higher in women than in men. From the 1950s until the present you will find the use of outpatient facilities and physicians' visits much higher in women than in men. If medical care was slowly improving after World War II in the United States women would have taken more advantage of medical services than men. I would also pose the hypothesis that coronary mortality in men rose after World War II because of increases in cigarette smoking. Women did not follow the pattern of men until more recently and, as yet, still do not smoke cigarettes at the same frequency or in the same quantity as men. Perhaps two patterns are occurring: for men, the rates rose with increased cigarette smoking and for women they declined because of their use of better medical care.

Oliver
Is there any evidence in the last decade that a different pattern is now developing as women are smoking more?

Haynes
We have some evidence that lung cancer mortality is rising in women in the United States. If lung cancer rates precede coronary heart disease mortality rates, there might be an increase in the latter in the next few years.

Epstein
Despite all the disparities, there is a parallel between changes in men and women. The decline in women in heart disease is less in countries where the increase in men is greatest, pointing to environmental factors that affect women and men similarly.

6

Wynn

How accurate do you think the national statistics are? It seems extraordinary that coronary heart disease mortality in a country like France or Spain should be so much lower than in England.

Epstein

Dr J. Richard in Paris has presented data from myocardial infarction registers in France which have also shown very low rates. We cannot explain some of these differences within Europe.

Beaumont J.-L.

The life expectancy in France is approximately the same as in other European countries.

Sternby

There are no good pathoanatomical studies on atherosclerosis in France. The International Atherosclerosis Project covered a large part of the world but left France out.

Epstein

Even if it was found in a reasonably large autopsy series in France that coronary atherosclerosis was less frequent, would one have much confidence in such data? At best they would point in one direction or other.

Robertson

Why are the rates of death from coronary heart disease so high in white South Africans? White South Africans would not seem to be socially deprived and it would not be easy to invoke that as a reason for their very high coronary rates. There are quite a lot of people in South Africa of British, indeed of Scottish, descent. There is a majority of Afrikaners and there is a high proportion of Jews. The Jewish population in white South Africa has a high death rate from coronary heart disease, while the people of British origin have lower rates than those of white Afrikaners.

Epstein

The south African data were not on the tape that was available to us. Rates are extraordinarily high in South Africa. There is a suggestion that type II hypercholesterolaemia is quite common among South Africans. I cannot imagine that this would account for all of the excessively high mortality from coronary heart disease.

Slack

In South Africa the coronary death rate is highest in the Afrikaners, and then marginally higher among those of Jewish than those of English extraction. The homozygotes for familial cholesterolaemia mainly appear in Afrikaner families and the calculations that I have done suggest that the heterozygote frequency of familial hypercholesterolaemia in the Afrikaners is as high as 1 in 80. It is probably about 1 in 500 among most other populations in the world. That condition is probably contributing to as many as 1 in 8 of the deaths from myocardial infarction in the Afrikaners under the age of 55. Those calculations were based on the Hardy-Weinberg equation and they are being borne out by epidemiological studies that we set up at that time. I think this does account for the peculiar situation in South Africa.

Nikkilä
In countries with a low sex ratio, close to 1, we may be dealing with a different disease. The risk factors may be quite different in these countries compared with countries where you have a high sex ratio. You might have another form of coronary heart disease which also results in coronary obstruction but which is unrelated to the major risk factors including the sex. Infection might be one possibility.

Epstein
Personally, I should not have thought so.

2. Genetic influences on coronary heart disease in women

J. Slack

The fundamental difference between men and women is genetic and is determined by the presence or absence of the Y chromosome. Among other manifestations of this difference there is a major difference in coronary death rates between men and women. At a meeting held in Edinburgh, reported in 1978,[1] it was recognised that in England and Wales coronary mortality rises inexorably with age in both men and women but throughout their lives the risks to men are greater than the risks to women and contrary to old rumours, there is no sudden departure from this pattern after the menopause (Fig. 2.1A).

Figure 2.1B shows this relationship in more detail; using the published death rates from the mid 1970s, there was a nearly sixfold difference in risk between men and women at age 55 with a gradual diminution in this ratio with increasing age until at 80 there is about double the risk of coronary death in men compared with women.

If there is a genetic contribution to the liability for death from coronary heart disease (CHD) the pattern of risk within families is now predictable. If a condition caused by several factors, some of which may be genetic, is less frequent in one sex then the relatives of the opposite sex will be more susceptible because there is likely to be a greater genetic component to their liability. Mrs Evans and I found this to be true for CHD when we studied the families of affected men and women in 1966[1] (Table 2.1).

When we looked at the risks to relatives of male patients who had sustained their first myocardial infarction under the age of 55 we found that the risk of coronary death to their male relatives under 55 was five times that of the general population, but the risk to their female relatives was not significantly increased; for the relatives of female patients who sustained their first myocardial infarction under the age of 55 we found that the risk of coronary death to their male relatives under 55 was five times that of the general population, but the risk to their female relatives was not significantly increased; for the relatives of female patients who sustained their first infarction under 55 the risk to their male relatives was nine times greater than that expected of the general population, and the risk to their female relatives was 4.5 times that of the general population. For women with myocardial infarction under 65 the risk to their male relatives was increased sixfold but among older women the genetic component seems to diminish.

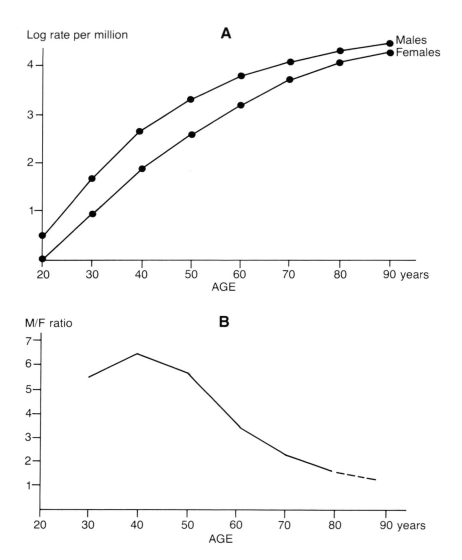

Fig. 2.1 A. Deaths from acute myocardial infarction in England and Wales. Classification 410. Registrar General 1973. B. Male/female ratio of deaths from acute myocardial infarction. Registrar General's statistics, England and Wales, 1973. Classification 410

Table 2.1 Increased risk of early coronary death in first-degree relatives of index patients with coronary heart disease under 55 years (Slack and Evans 1966).

	Male patients under 55
Male relatives under 55	5.16**
Female relatives under 65	2.75
	Female patients under 55
Male relatives under 55	9.01**
Female relatives under 65	4.62*

*p<0.01>0.001, **p<0.001

These family studies do not, of course, distinguish whether the liability within families is due to the common family environment such as the parental smoking habits or the quality of the home cooking or to the shared family genes. To examine the genetic component it is necessary to turn to human twin-studies and in 1970 I did this with Harvald and Hauge, who had maintained the comprehensive Danish twin-study for a considerable period[1] (Table 2.2).

Table 2.2 Concordance rates for coronary heart disease in twins.

Sex		Zygosity	Concordance rate Numbers		Significance of difference in concordance rate
♂ ♂		MZ	30/77	0.39	p<0.05
		DZ	32/122	0.26	
♀ ♂		MZ	12/27	0.44	p<0.01
		DZ	8/54	0.14	
♂ ♀	DZ	probands	7/53	0.13	
	DZ	probands	8/19	0.43	

There we found that for 77 male monozygous twins the concordance rate was 0.39, significantly greater than for 122 dizygous male twins. For 27 pairs of female monozygous twins the concordance rate was 0.44, while for 54 pairs of dizygous female twins the concordance rate was 0.14. A little more evidence for this trend was provided by the differences in the unlike sex twins where an affected male provided a concordance rate of only 0.13 while an affected female provided a concordance rate of 0.43. These differences, imperfect though human breeding and rearing experiments must be, do suggest that there *is* a substantial genetic component to the liability to CHD and that the genetic component is predictably greater in women than in men.

Using Falconer's model to calculate the heritability of CHD from our family studies it may be estimated that genetic factors may be contributing 60% of the total variation in liability to CHD in men under 55 years and as much as 80% of the variation in women of the same age. The calculations apply only to the population we have studied, not to all men and women. It is also possible that a common family environment may be causing an overestimate in the family studies, but its contribution is likely to be small in a condition which occurs at an age when families have split up for some considerable length of time.

It now becomes necessary to ask what the components of the inherited liability to CHD are and how much each component contributes to the variation of the liability. Looking at the established risk factors such as smoking, serum cholesterol concentration and blood pressure it is possible to examine the evidence for a genetic component and to calculate what contribution the component might make to the total liability.

I can make no useful comment about genetic influences on family smoking habits. The National Pooling Project showed that systolic blood pressure in middle-aged men was an important risk factor and Miall's[1] family study of blood pressure contains suitable information to investigate family similarities (Table 2.3). There was no significant correlation between man and wife. The correlation between father and son was negligible and the highest correlation was observed between mother and daughter. We have to go back to 1930 to find reports on a twin-study for systolic blood pressure by Percy Stocks[1] and I have used his data and Charles Smith's method to estimate the heritability of systolic blood pressure and the possible contribution of common family environment (Table 2.4). He found the correlation between monozygous twins was 0.69, giving a heritability of 69% with a small and acceptable standard error of five. The correlation between dizygous twins was 0.32 giving a heritability of 64% with a considerably larger standard error, but the similarity between these two figures suggests a small contribution from common family environment, and this is supported by the final calculation using Falconer's method which gives an estimated heritability for systolic blood pressure among these Welsh twins of 74%.

Table 2.3 Parent/child correlations for age-adjusted systolic blood pressure (Miall et al 1967).

	n	r
Father/son	132	0.14
Father/daughter	137	0.22
Mother/son	129	0.20
Mother/daughter	140	0.41
Spouse	130	0.009

Table 2.4 Heritability of systolic blood pressure from Welsh twin-study from Percy Stocks (1930).

	% Heritability $\pm$ 1 SE
r	69 $\pm$ 5
$2r_{DZ}$	64 $\pm$ 20
$2(r_{MZ} \quad r_{DZ})$	74 $\pm$ 22.4

I have found no useful family or twin-studies of British twins which allow estimates for heritability of serum cholesterol concentration. Family studies reported by Adlersberg[1] from the United States in 1957 showed within family correlations which were negligible between spouses, small between father and son and, as for systolic blood pressure, greatest between mother and daughter (Table 2.5).

Table 2.5 Parent/child correlations for age-adjusted serum cholesterol concentrations (Adlersberg 1957).

	n	r
Father/son	181	0.16
Father/daughter	192	0.26
Mother/son	181	0.34
Mother/daughter	192	0.39
Spouse	201	0.006

Twin-studies of serum cholesterol concentration has been rather unsatisfactory, partly because of relatively small numbers and partly because of unexplained differences in variance which prohibit calculations of heritability from correlations. I have therefore used Pikkarainen's[1] twin-study of serum cholesterol in male twins to show estimates of heritability which allow for comparisons with my estimates of heritability of systolic blood pressure but are certainly not ideal (Table 2.6). He found a correlation of 0.56 for serum cholesterol concentration in monozygous twins giving an estimated heritability of 56% with an acceptable standard error of nine. He found a correlation of 0.37 in dizygous twins giving an estimated heritability of 74%. The discrepancy between these two estimates suggests a strong contribution from common family environment and this is supported by the lower heritability estimate from Falconer's calculation of 38%, which is probably more accurate in spite of the large standard error produced by the more sophisticated calculation.

Table 2.6 Heritability of serum cholesterol from Finnish twin-study calculated from Pikkarainen (1966).

	% Heritability $\pm$ 1 SE
r_{MZ}	56 ± 9
$2r_{DZ}$	74 ± 24
$2(r_{MZ} - r_{DZ})$	38 ± 30

In Table 2.7 I have attempted to calculate the effect of the heritability estimates on the blood pressure of male relatives who might be at risk of CHD because their mothers or sisters have had myocardial infarctions.[1] By sleight of hand, and probably quite illegally, I have changed from systolic to diastolic blood pressure but, though you may not forgive me, you will see my reason for this in a moment.

Table 2.7 Mean diastolic blood pressure (BP) and serum cholesterol concentration in first-degree relatives of index patients at 50 years.

	Diastolic BP mm Hg	Serum cholesterol mmol/l
Female patient	112.8 (2 SD)	8.6 (2 SD)
Male 1st° Rel.	94.5	5.8
Inc. Risk	×1.2	×1.3
Female 1st° Rel.	93.7	6.5

Let us suppose a woman of 50 has a myocardial infarction and her blood pressure is raised 2 standard deviations above the population mean. If the heritability of diastolic blood pressure is 70% then the blood pressure of male and female first-degree relatives of the woman patient are expected on average to be 94.5 and 93.7 respectively. Similarly, the serum cholesterol concentrations of male and female first-degree relatives of a woman who has a myocardial infarction with a serum cholesterol concentration raised by 2 standard deviations above the mean can be expected, on average, to have serum cholesterol concentrations of 6.6 and 6.5 mmol/l. Even with such high and obvious risk factors the estimated heritabilities of blood pressure and serum cholesterol do not have a devastatingly great effect on the relatives. If this effect is examined in the light of the possible increased risk calculated from Stamler's National Pooling Project in 1970 the relative risk to the male relatives of the hypertensive women is 1.2 and the relative risk to the male relatives of the hypercholesterolaemic woman is 1.3—provided, of course, that her myocardial infarction was associated with a polygenic system of liability and not with a dominantly inherited condition. Whether these calculations are accurate or not it is clear to me that the inheritance of the recognised risk factors is not sufficient to account for the observed increase in the risk of coronary death in the relatives of young women with myocardial infarction.

Other risk factors such as the thrombotic factors are emerging. It will be very interesting to see whether they are shown to be inherited characteristics and, if so, whether they are so strongly inherited that they can account for the remaining risk within families—especially of female patients.

Perhaps it is time now to look afresh at the differences between men and women and to look for some other clues about the difference in risk between the sexes. I have explained that the difference between the sexes is genetic and the fundamental difference lies in the presence or absence of the Y chromosome. If the Y chromosome is present you are a boy. If there are one, two, three or more X chromosomes present in the absence of a Y, you are a girl. Now the coronary mortality in women with two X chromosomes is about 10 years delayed compared with the male with one X and one Y chromosome. This relationship persists even in heterozygotes for familial hypercholesterolaemia where hypercholesterolaemia is acting as an overwhelming risk factor. The temptation is to suggest that the extra X chromosome and accompanying increased female sex hormones act as a protective mechanism in normal females.

Since accurate karyotyping has been available it has been possible to identify individuals with aberrant sex chromosomes who can provide a natural variation in the number of X and Y chromosomes. A recent report by Price and Clayton[2] from Edinburgh compared the coronary mortality in men with Klinefelter's syndrome— that is, men with two X chromosomes and one Y—with the coronary mortality in normal men. There were 6419 man years at risk among the men with Klinefelter's syndrome and there were 17 deaths from coronary artery disease. Over the same period, 18.7 deaths might have been expected from men in the general population— a difference that was clearly not statistically significant. I understand from Dr Price that the men did not differ from the normal male population in their smoking habits, blood pressure or serum cholesterol concentrations (personal communication). Men with Klinefelter's are known to have increased plasma oestrogen levels but their testosterone levels have been reported as variable. Information about coronary mortality in other sex chromosome abnormalities—such as women with one X chromosome, Turner's syndrome, or men with two chromosomes, the XYY syndrome—as far as I know are not available.

Embryologically the fetus starts with undifferentiated gonads. If the Y chromosome is present the testes are formed and an ovary is formed if the Y chromosome is absent. In the male fetus the testes secrete fetal androgen and testosterone which stimulate the Wolffian ducts to develop into male internal and external genitalia. The fetal ovary secretes neither testosterone nor the factor necessary to inhibit the development of the Mullerian structures and a normal female with uterus and fallopian tubes is born.

Since the Klinefelter's male with the extra X chromosome and increased oestrogen levels has the coronary mortality of a normal male it suggests that, rather than a protective effect of the X chromosome or female sex hormones, there is an aggressive effect of the Y which may be acting through the presence of the male hormones. I found no information available about the state of the coronary vessels of virilised females, but I did find a paper which reported the life expectancy of castrated males.

In 1969 Hamilton and Mestler[3] reported an account of the life span of eunuchs who had been castrated in an institution in the United States. The life expectancy of the groups of castrated and non-castrated patients were compared. The youngest being castrated at 8 years of age and the oldest at 59. The mean age at death of the eunuchs was significantly higher than the mean age of the intact men, their mean life span being 13.5 years longer than the intact males and not significantly different from the expected life span of the female institutionalised patients. The life span of the eunuchs seemed greatest in those castrated before 15 years of age.

I would not like to suggest that too much should be deduced from these observations, but the experiment is never likely to be repeated. It will be difficult to collect information about coronary mortality in Turner's syndrome since most girls diagnosed will receive hormone treatment from adolescence onwards. It may, however, be possible to obtain some information about the life span of men with the XYY syndrome and perhaps we shall hear more about the coronary vessels of virilised women.

Meanwhile, the genetic contribution to coronary death which can be handed on from an affected woman is difficult to attribute entirely to the conventional recognised risk factors and it is not clear to me whether the difference in coronary mortality between men and women should be attributed to a protection of the X or the aggression of the Y chromosome.

SUMMARY

The difference in risk of death from CHD between men and women predicts that if there is a genetic component to liability to coronary death the risk to relatives of affected women will be greater than to those of affected men. This hypothesis has been confirmed by family studies and studies of twins confirm that there is a genetic contribution to the liability to coronary death which is greater in female patients.

The pattern of inheritance of recognised risk factors for CHD is mainly polygenic and, except for families with familial hypercholesterolaemia, the inheritance of serum cholesterol concentration or hypertension does not account for the observed increased risk of coronary death within families of affected patients.

The reason for lower coronary mortality in women is not clear. An extra X chromosome in men with Klinefelter's syndrome fails to protect them from the coronary death rate of normal men. It is possible that the Y chromosome causes an added risk through the production of androgens from the male gonads.

REFERENCES

[1]Oliver M F. Coronary heart disease in young women. Edinburgh, London, New York: Churchill Livingstone, 1978
[2]Price W H, Clayton J F. Oestrogens and coronary artery disease in men. Lancet 1983; 2: 860–1
[3]Hamilton J B, Mestler G E. Mortality and survival: comparison of eunuchs with intact men and women in mentally retarded population. J Gerontol 1969; 24: 395–411

Discussion on chapter 2

Rifkind
I wonder whether the lipid or lipoprotein levels of Klinefelter's syndrome were known in contrast to normal man?

Slack
I don't know if the HDL cholesterol level is abnormal in Klinefelter's syndrome.

Wynn
Is testosterone the fatal factor in the male? The castrated males survived longer but the Klinefelter males did not, despite the higher oestrogen levels?

Slack
Yes.

Oliver
There are three studies in the literature reporting the relative freedom of coronary arterial and aortic disease in patients treated with large doses of oestrogen for cancer of the prostate.

Beaumont J.-L.
I would like to give you information on skin differences between men and women with respect to skin cholesterol content. In well-defined type IIa hypercholestero-laemia men and women had no great difference in blood cholesterol, HDL and LDL, but female skin contained more cholesterol ester and had a higher CE/FC ratio. In normal men and women the CD/FC ratio is higher compared with type IIa patients in both sexes. Through certain pharmacological manipulation in pe IIa patients, the EC fraction and the EC/FC ratio increases in both sexes but more so in men. Our ongoing studies support the theory that the difference between men and women has to do with the balance of EC and FC in the cells.

Oliver
In 1953 the late George Boyd and I[1] found that free cholesterol did not change at all during the menstrual cycle whereas there was a striking fall in ester cholesterol and total cholesterol at the time of ovulation. This was a sharp and short fall lasting for less than 24 hours and the reduction was of the order of 12% from the preovulatory phase and in the postovulatory phase the ester cholesterol rose by about 15%. Thus there is a regular fluctuation in ester cholesterol which is not present in free cholesterol.

Haynes
A number of investigators have suggested that menstrual periods in women may have some benefit and may explain some of the coronary differences between men and women.

Slack
Haemoglobin is lower in women—perhaps as a result of the menstrual periods. I

believe that serum cholesterol is weakly correlated with haemoglobin levels, so the temptation is to suggest that serum cholesterol concentration is periodically lower in women. The cholesterol does not really seem to be acting as a very strong risk factor in women. Taking the Framingham study, many years of investigation were needed to show the weak connection between serum cholesterol concentration and the risk of female coronary artery disease. So I don't really believe that the connection between menstruation and the possibility of reducing coronary risk by causing anaemia would be very strong, but it is the best explanation I can offer.

Shapiro
We should not take the failure of Framingham to show a relationship between cholesterol and risk in females too seriously. The numbers were inadequate.

Rosenberg
We have found that in younger women cholesterol stands out strongly, particularly below the age of 50.

Slack
Are you sure that they did not have familial hypocholesterolaemia?

Rosenberg
It seems very unlikely that this would explain it. Also in regard to haematocrit, which we were discussing before, we have recorded haematocrit and haemoglobin levels in our study of young men and related these to the risk of myocardial infarction. Preliminary analyses show that there is no relationship.

de Faire
We have performed studies on families of myocardial infarction patients who have had their infarct before the age of 45, and it seems as if the genetic component is stronger among males than females. Segregation analyses and pathway analyses were used.

Robertson
We should remember that there is no difficulty in finding young women with coronary heart disease if you take those young women who present with severe hypertension.

REFERENCE

[1]Oliver M F, Boyd G S. Changes in plasma lipids during menstrual cycle. Clin Sci 1953; 12: 217-22

3. Familial occurrence of coronary heart disease and major risk factors

A.M. Rissanen

FAMILIAL OCCURRENCE OF CORONARY HEART DISEASE

Frequency of coronary heart disease in relatives of patients and controls

Most of the evidence of a familial component in coronary heart disease (CHD) comes from studies comparing the frequency of the disease in relatives of CHD patients with controls. These studies have uniformly demonstrated a greater frequency of the disease in the relatives of patients,[1] but the strength of the familial aggregation varies widely, reflecting the remarkable variety of the patients studied and the methods used. This heterogeneity is evident in Table 3.1, which summarises the pertinent features of the major case-control studies of CHD.

Parents
The frequency of CHD found in parents of patients has, in general, been about twice as great as that in parents of controls (Table 3.1). While distinct in fathers of male patients,[2-8,11-13] especially in those of young cases,[3,5,13] the aggregation of the disease usually has been negligible in the mothers of CHD patients.[2,5,6,11] Nevertheless, some excess of either CHD [3,4,12,13] or of cerebrovascular accidents [5,13] in mothers of young patients has been reported. The aggregation of CHD in mothers is slightly more apparent in the few studies in which there are female patients among the cases.[4,7,10]

Siblings
The degree of familial aggregation of CHD found among siblings of male cases exceeds that observed among their parents in most,[2-4,6,8,9,11-14] but not in all,[5,7] studies in which comparable information on the occurrence of the disease in both parents and siblings has been given (Table 3.1). The aggregation seems to be more pronounced for the brothers than for the sisters of patients.[3,7-9,11-13] The relative risk of CHD for siblings of patients has varied considerably, ranging from virtually no excess to more than tenfold excesses when compared with the risks for control siblings. Such variation in risk may largely result from the wide age range of the cases. The risk of the disease is greatest for the sibs of the youngest CHD patients.[3,13,15] In a study of families of men with myocardial infarction (MI) from South and

18

East Finland, for instance, a steep gradient of risk of CHD for the sibs according to the age of the patient was-demonstrated (Fig. 3.1).[13] Depending on whether the diagnosis of MI in the patient had first been established before the age of 46, at age 46–50, or at age 51–55 years, the risk of having the disease by the age of 55 was, respectively, 11.4, 8.3 and 1.3 times greater in the South and 6.7, 3.6 and 1.8 times greater in the East for the brothers of patients than for the brothers of controls. The prevalence of CHD among the relatives of the youngest patients in South Finland was similar to the high incidence area of East Finland (as opposed to differences observed between the two areas for relatives of older patients), suggesting that genetic determination of the disease in the very young was strong enough to outweigh any regional differences in environmental risk factors.

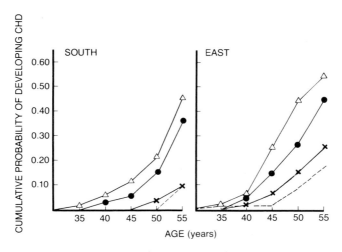

Fig. 3.1 Cumulative probalility of developing fatal or non-fatal CHD for the brothers of the probands whose first myocardial infarction was diagnosed before age 46 (Δ), at age 46–50 (●), or at age 50–55 (x), and for the brothers of reference men (---). From Rissanen[13]

Relatively little is known about the aggregation of CHD in siblings of female patients.[10] We recently completed a study on the occurrence of CHD in the families of 121 female and 586 male survivors of MI (Liskola et al, to be published.) These patients were participants in the coronary rehabilitation courses of the Social Insurance Institute in Finland. CHD was more common among the sibs of the female patients than among those of the male patients. The disease was reported in 10.7% and 5.2% of the sisters as well as in 23.8% and 18.3% of the brothers of the female and male patients, respectively. The risk of CHD was greater for the sibs of both female and male patients with the first MI before age 50 than for the sibs of patients who had MI first at a later age.

First- and second-degree relatives
In the studies reporting CHD among first-degree relatives,[7,14,16-19] two-to fivefold excess risks of CHD were found for male first-degree relatives of male patients. Somewhat contradicting the low risks reported for mothers and sisters separately, the overall risks for the female first-degree relatives of male patients were also found

Table 3.1 Occurrence of coronary heart disease (CHD) in parents and siblings of patients and controls (selected studies) MI=myocardial infarction, IHD=ischaemic heart disease, AP=angina pectoris.

Source		Parents (%)		Sibs affected		Methodological notes	
		Fathers	Mothers	Brothers	Sisters	Definition of CHD in relatives	Patients cases and controls
Gertler and White[2]	Patient	37.1	9.8	8.6		Reported CHD death	97 male survivors of definite MI, age ≤40. Absence of diabetes and hypertension
	Control	18.5	7.7	1.0			146 age-matched healthy control men
Shanoff et al[3]	Patient age 30–50	61.7	40.0	12.2	3.0	Reported CHD, fatal or non-fatal	102 male survivors of MI, age 30–70. Absence of diabetes and hypertension
	age 51–70	25.0	23.3				
	Control	29.6	19.8	1.2	0.7		100 hospitalised control men, age 30–70
Rose[4]	Patient	20.0	13.3	2.9		Reported IHD death	65 male and 10 female survivors of MI, age ≤70. 75 hospitalised age- and sex-matched controls
	Control	10.7	4.0	0.8			
Phillips et al[5]	Patient age ≤52	19.3	8.4	8.2		CHD in death certificate (parents) or in death certificate or hospital record (sibs)	264 men with MI (non-fatal, fatal or silent), or AP, age 45–65, from a population study
	age 53–64	13.8	13.1	3.9			
	Control	6.1	8.3	5.3			264 age-matched pairs from the same population
Welin[6]	Patient	16.3	5.8	4.9		Reported MI, fatal or non-fatal	26 male survivors of MI aged 50 or 60 from a population study
	Control	11.7	6.3	1.8			A population sample of 969 men, aged 50 or 60, free of clinical CHD

Table 3.1 (cont).

Source		Parents Fathers	Mothers %	Sibs Brothers	Sisters affected	Methodological notes Definition of CHD in relatives	Patients cases and controls
Thordarsson and Fridriksson[7]	Patient	31.4	16.5	24.2	18.1	IHD in death certificate	108 male and 42 female survivors of MI, age ≤70
	Control	18.4	10.5	17.8	13.7		150 age- and sex-matched controls, no awareness of CHD
Rissanen[8]	Patient	24.5	12.3	28.6	10.6	Parents: CHD before age 70 in death certificate	309 men with AP, or fatal/non-fatal MI, age ≤55
	Control	8.0	7.6	7.9	5.3	Siblings: CHD in death certificate or disease records	106 age- and sex-matched controls, free of clinical CHD
Hamby[9]	Patient	56.8		23.6	5.9	Reported CHD, confirmed by another family member	411 men with symptoms of CHD and positive angiogram
	Control	40.2		1.9	1.2		184 men with other heart diseases and negative angiogram
Rosenberg et al[10]	Patient	15.3	9.4	9.4		Reported MI or stroke before age 60	255 female survivors of MI, age ≤50
	Control	14.0	6.4	5.6			802 hospitalised age-matched women

to be distinctly increased. For instance, in the most careful study of its kind, Slack and Evans in 1966[16] reported that compared with the general population the male and female first-degree relatives of male coronary patients under age 55 carried, respectively, fivefold and 2.5-fold increases in the risk of dying from CHD by age 55. The risks were greatest for the youngest relatives of the youngest patients, especially of the female patients. This finding points to a more conspicuous familial component in CHD of women than of men. A striking heritable component for CHD that is transmitted through the maternal line of inheritance was also suggested by Icelandic investigators who reported an extraordinarily high mortality from CHD for maternal uncles and aunts of coronary patients.[7] The mortality was not remarkable in other second-degree relatives.

Comments on methodology
Studies on familial occurrence of CHD are beset with a number of problems.[20-21] These are compounded in case-control studies of familial aggregation. It is difficult to diagnose CHD in a person available for examination; diagnosing it in a person long ago deceased or beyond reach is, at best, hazardous. Reports of disease in such persons, usually obtained from index patients and controls, may be grossly inaccurate. It is also clear that index patients with CHD have a better recall of similar diseases in the family than do healthy controls. Moreover, if the index patients are selected from hospitals rather than from the population at large, the distinct chance remains that an excess of patients from families with several affected members enter the study as index cases. Many case-control studies with the biases listed above may end up overestimating the strength of familial aggregation of CHD. On the other hand, case-control comparisons including CHD events of young and old relatives alike underestimate the strength of the familial component, which probably is confined only to early events. Some of the methodological weaknesses discussed above may be avoided in studies on the familial occurrence of CHD in the general population.

Familial occurrence of CHD in population studies

Parental and family history as predictors of CHD risk
The relation of family history to the incidence of CHD was investigated in the Western Collaborative Group study.[22] The incidence of CHD among men who reported a parental history of the disease was found to be about twice as great as that among men reporting no such history. Because of the unreliability of the reported parental histories of CHD,[6] the disease experience of the offspring has also been analysed in relation to the less questionable reports on parental age at death. [6,23] These studies have shown that early parental death, irrespective of cause, predisposes young men to death from CHD to an essentially similar extent as does a reported parental death from CHD, all ages considered.[23] According to a Swedish investigation,[6] a history of parental death at an early age from any cause may be a better predictor of risk than is a history of CHD death at any age. Much of the excess risk found to be associated with early parental death from any cause may, however, be attributable to early CHD, which is the primary or contributory cause to many of the early deaths.

A considerably greater predictive power for early than late parental deaths from CHD was suggested by the findings of the Tecumseh Community Study, the first prospective survey primarily designed to assess the role of familial factors in CHD. [20,24-26] In a report published in 1970[26] it was shown that within a follow-up period of about 4 years 12.8% of the initially well men aged 40–59 reporting a paternal death from CHD before age 65 had also died of CHD. Only 3.2% of the men reporting a paternal death from CHD at a later age, and a mere 0.7% of the men reporting a paternal death from other causes, had died of CHD. A somewhat similar trend was observed with regard to maternal mortality. The incidence of non-fatal CHD, on the other hand, was highest among men whose parents had died of CHD after age 65 rather than earlier. These results suggest that the familial determinants of fatal and non-fatal CHD may differ.

Sibship aggregation of CHD
The concordance of CHD within sibships was investigated in the Framingham Offspring Study.[27] During a 26 year follow-up the incidence of MI in initially well brother pairs was about twice that expected, but it was not higher than expected within sister pairs. The number of new cases in this analysis, however, was fairly small despite the large base population and long observation period. A unique approach for the study of familial CHD has been adopted in the Utah Pedigree Study,[28] which is based on the genealogical data available for a large proportion of the state's Mormon residents. A preliminary report[28] showed that brother-pair aggregation for coronary deaths was 7.7 times greater than expected and that half of all early heart attacks were concentrated in 5% of the families.

Spouse concordance for CHD
CHD tends to aggregate not only in blood relatives but also in unrelated family members such as spouses. The concordance for CHD among spouses was first suggested by the elaborate studies of Thomas and Cohen.[29] These findings were confirmed in the Framingham population.[30] The risk of the wife dying from CHD has been found to be greatest in the few months after the coronary death of the husband. The spousal concordance for CHD may reflect both the stress imposed on the family and contribution of shared environmental influences.

Twin-studies of CHD
Twin-studies are one of the best means available at present for assessing the role of hereditary versus environmental factors in the causation of disease. Several studies, notable among them those from the Scandinavian twin registries, have revealed a higher concordance rate for CHD in monozygotic than in dizygotic pairs.[1] In the Danish registry,[31] for instance, the concordance for fatal coronary occlusion was reported to be greater in monozygotic than in dizygotic pairs, especially in the female pairs. Furthermore, the concordance in the unlike sexed pairs of female probands was greater than in those of male probands. These findings suggest a considerable genetic determination of CHD, particularly in women. In the Swedish registry,[32] the coincidence rate of coronary deaths in monozygotic pairs was greater than in dizygotic pairs during a follow-up period from 1962–73. The coincidence rates among the monozygotic twins born in 1901–25 were six times greater than

those among the monozygotic pairs born in 1889–1900. These observations are the most cogent evidence available today of a stronger genetic component in early onset CHD than in late onset disease.

Familial occurrence of major coronary risk factors in relation to CHD

Hypertension
The familial component in blood pressure is well documented.[37,38] There is a positive correlation between the blood pressure levels of family members, and this similarity is greater between relatives than between unrelated people sharing the same household. Hypertension and high blood pressure levels aggregate in families and normotensive members of such families may show signs of disturbed blood pressure regulation.[38] Some of these signs, such as abnormal cation fluxes in cell membranes, may come to serve as genetic markers for some forms of hypertension.[38,39] Both genes and shared environment contribute to the observed familial resemblance in blood pressure. Tests of heritability usually show strong genetic effects suggesting that up to half the population variance of blood pressure may be due to genetic factors.

Several lines of evidence suggest that the familial aggregation of high blood pressure is associated with the familial occurrence of CHD. Raised blood pressure levels and an excess number of hypertensives have been found among relatives of coronary patients, [8,11,13,40,41] in surviving co-twins in pairs discordant for CHD death,[32] and in people with a family history of CHD or cardiovascular disease. [6,29,42,43] Conversely, young and middle-aged individuals with high blood pressure have been reported to have an increased parental mortality from early CHD, the most distinct excess mortality being among the mothers of women with high blood pressure.[25] Other studies also suggest particular involvement of the maternal line of inheritance in the association between familial CHD and hypertension. Hypertension is more common in coronary patients whose mother (rather than father) died of premature CHD.[9,13] Furthermore, a maternal (but not a paternal) history of hypertension and stroke has been shown to be associated with an enhanced risk of CHD in the offspring, as evidenced by higher than normal blood pressure, body weight and serum triglycerides, and lowered high-density lipoprotein (HDL) levels.[44] Other studies, however, show a limited association or no association between family history of CHD and blood pressure level. [17,18,22,45]

Lipoprotein disturbances
The importance of genetic factors in the variation in serum lipid and lipoprotein levels is well established. [1,45] Serum total cholesterol, total triglyceride and various lipoprotein concentrations are correlated in first-degree relatives and in twins, but usually not in spouses or in adopted children and their parents. The variation of serum lipoprotein and lipid levels in the population at large is determined by both genetic and environmental factors, and by their interaction. Genetic influences are most conspicuous at the upper end of the population distribution of the serum lipoprotein and lipid values (in the so-called hyperlipoproteinaemias). These influences are usually polygenic, but are occasionally primarily determined by a single gene.

24

Familial hyperlipoproteinaemias

Familial monogenic hypercholesterolaemia, the most thoroughly investigated form of familial hyperlipoproteinaemia, is caused by one of several mutations in the gene specifying the low-density lipoprotein (LDL) receptor.[47] Appreciably raised LDL concentrations caused by this disorder occur at an estimated frequency of one per 200–500. Most homozygotes die of CHD before the age of 30. For heterozygotes the risk of CHD by middle-age is increased 10–25-fold for the men, and somewhat less for the women. The pattern of CHD is quite consistent within a family affected by monozygotic familial hypercholesterolaemia, but varies from one family to another according to the variability in the level of the LDL concentrations and other risk factors. Despite its high atherogenicity, familial monogenic hypercholesterolaemia probably contributes little to the population risk of CHD. It has been encountered in only 2–6% of young male survivors of MI.[48,49] Even so, its frequency in male patients with other forms of CHD and in female coronary patients remains to be established.

Hypercholesterolaemia, hypertriglyceridaemia, or both, are characteristic of members of families affected by familial multiple lipoprotein type hyperlipidaemia.[48] An increased risk of early CHD is well established in this genetically heterogeneous disorder, which was encountered in about a quarter of the young male survivors of MI in Helsinki.[48] This abnormality appears to be the most common form of familial hyperlipidaemia in young male survivors of MI. [45,48,49]

Premature atherosclerosis is common in the rare familial type 3 hyperlipoproteinaemia,[50] which was encountered with certainty in one and possibly in three others of the 500 male survivors of MI under age 60 in Seattle.[49] Very rare type 5 familial hyperlipoproteinaemia is associated with an increased risk of CHD, with rates of 1–2% reported among coronary patients.[51] Some, but perhaps not all, forms of familial hypertriglyceridaemia may carry an increased risk of CHD.[52] This abnormality was found in 5% of the male survivors of MI in Seattle but less frequently in Helsinki.[48,49]

The assessment of the contribution of polygenic hyperlipoproteinaemias to the familial liability to CHD is hampered by the lack of accurate diagnostic criteria for these disorders. In view of its high population frequency, polygenic (LDL-) hypercholesterolaemia can be expected to be strongly related to the familial occurrence of CHD. An increased prevalence of hypercholesterolaemia of other than the monogenic type is a frequent finding in survivors of MI and in their relatives, [48,49,53] including children.[54]

Several sources of evidence suggest that the familial aggregation of high levels of serum total and LDL-cholesterol, irrespective of cause, are associated with the familial occurrence of CHD. Thus, the rate of premature CHD is increased in parents of both children[54–56] and adults[25] with the highest serum cholesterol levels. Conversely, the serum total cholesterol or LDL-cholesterol concentration have frequently [13,41,48,49,57–59] but not invariably[60] been found to be raised in the relatives of young coronary patients with an almost fourfold enrichment of hypercholesterolaemia in the offspring of young male survivors of MI.[61] Furthermore, a family history of CHD has been reported to be associated with increased serum total cholesterol and LDL-cholesterol levels in middle-aged people. [6,18,22,29,44]

Serum triglycerides are raised in coronary patients and their adult relatives alike. [13,41,48,49,57–59] Increased levels of serum triglycerides have been found also in people with a family history of CHD in some [6,43,60] but not in all [18,22] studies. Relatives of hypertriglyceridaemic children have not been reported to have an increased mortality from CHD. [56,62]

High-density lipoproteins

Like other serum lipoproteins, the quantity and quality of HDL is subject to genetic and environmental control. Raised levels of HDL-cholesterol which may occasionally be transmitted as an autosomal dominant trait are associated with a less than average rate of CHD and with an increased life expectancy. [63] Low levels of HDL-cholesterol, associated with an increased risk of the disease, have been found in children [64] and adult relatives [60] of patients with CHD, and in people with a family history of CHD. [65] HDL-cholesterol levels in schoolchildren have been shown to be better predictors of CHD in grandparents than total or LDL-cholesterol levels. [56]

Other familial risk factors

Diabetes

An inherited basis has been established for various types of diabetes. [66] Clinical diabetes, especially the non-insulin-dependent type, aggregates in families. The findings from the Tecumseh Community Study strongly suggested that familial aggregation of diabetes and CHD would be interconnected. The investigators reported both an increased mortality from premature CHD for parents of middle-aged subjects with high serum glucose levels, [25] and an increased prevalence of diabetes among the middle-aged offspring of parents who died of premature CHD. [26] An increased prevalence of diabetes or raised blood glucose levels [19,59] have been found among the relatives of coronary patients and in coronary patients with a maternal history [9] or strong family history [11] of CHD. Other studies have failed to show any convincing association between the familial occurrence of CHD and diabetes [22,32] or raised serum glucose levels, [41,45] but any association in these studies may well have been masked by methodological weaknesses. Hence, the relation between the familial aggregations of the two traits will require further study.

Obesity

Overweight and obesity tend to run in families. [67] There is little evidence of an association between the occurrence of obesity and CHD in families. As a rule male patients with CHD and their relatives are no more overweight, [6,11,22,29,32] but may be more mesomorphic, [2] than others. Offspring of overweight parents do not seem to carry a greater than usual risk of CHD. [29]

Smoking

To some extent smoking habits are familial. They tend to be similar in parents and their children [68] as well as in twins, especially in monozygotic pairs. [69] Spouses also resemble each other with regard to smoking. [70] In fact, this may be the coronary risk factor they share to the greatest degree.

The few studies giving data on the familial occurrence of CHD and smoking do not suggest a close association. Smoking habits have been found to be similar in relatives of coronary patients and controls[7,11] and in men with or without a family history of CHD.[6,18,22] Smoking patterns do not differ significantly between the surviving co-twins of pairs discordant for death from CHD and those discordant for death from other causes.[32]

Other lifestyle variables
Family members share a common physical and socioeconomic background. Some resemblance between relatives is therefore to be expected with regard to most personal characteristics and habits such as physical activity, diet and behaviour.[69] By their influence on the major risk factors or by other mechanisms, these familial similarities may enhance the familial susceptibility to CHD or decrease it.[71]

Contribution of risk factors to the familial susceptibility to CHD

Major risk factors
In the studies reviewed above, modest associations have been found between the familial occurrence of the established risk factors and CHD. The association has been somewhat more evident, however, in studies in which the joint contribution of several of the risk factors has been taken into account. Thus, parents of middle-aged men[72,73] and of children[54] with pronounced risk factor scores have been shown to have remarkably increased morbidity and mortality from CHD, especially at an early age.[26]

A series of studies on the families of Finnish men with CHD have shown a close association between the occurrence of CHD and its major risk factors.[8,11,13,57] Clustering of CHD within the relatives was almost invariably accompanied by familial clustering of hyperlipidaemia and/or hypertension, not only in the family members themselves affected by CHD but also in their younger sibs who as yet had shown no evidence of the disease. The association between the familial occurrence of CHD and its two major risk factors was most impressive in those families in which the mother had died of the disease at an early age. About half the daughters and sons of these women had both hypertension and hyperlipidaemia, suggesting that the affected mothers had passed on to their offspring potent determinants of early-onset hypertension and hyperlipidaemia. Several lines of evidence suggest that only part of the overall familial aggregation of CHD can be attributed to the familial aggregations of the major risk factors. No major differences have been found in risk factor levels of men with or without family or parental history of CHD.[14,17,28,44,45,74,75] However, in some of these studies, the association between family history and risk factors may have been weakened by the use of unconfirmed histories covering the clinically relevant early cases of CHD in the family and the less relevant late cases alike. Similarly, in several studies the concomitant effects of risk factors have been found to be too weak to account for the association observed between parental history and the occurrence of either symptomatic disease[18,22] or of angiographically proved CHD.[34] Likewise, the established risk factors explain only part of the higher frequency of CHD in the surviving co-twins whose partners died from CHD over the frequency in those whose partners died of other causes.[32] Moreover, the incidence of CHD in brother pairs in Framingham was shown to exceed that expected on the basis of the relatively strong contributions of the major risk factors.[27] It thus appears that part of the familial predisposition to CHD is mediated through as yet unidentified mechanisms. The contribution of the established risk factors may not, however, be similar in different ethnic groups, in different environments, at different ages, or in the different forms of CHD.[76]

Other possible factors
Some of the apoproteins of lipoproteins have been linked to atherosclerosis.[77] Apo B, the apoprotein of LDL, and apo A-I, the major apoprotein of HDL, are of particular interest, as both are strongly heritable[1] and strongly associated with premature CHD.[77] Familially determined increases in apo B and decreases in apo A-I levels may be expected to contribute significantly to the familial liability to CHD, but their contribution at present is unknown. Genetic polymorphisms of apoproteins, especially of apo E and of Lp(a)-lipoprotein may influence the risk of CHD.[1] The Lp(a)-lipoprotein is strongly heritable and strongly associated with clinical CHD, but the mechanisms behind the association are obscure. As Lp(a)-phenotype is inherited and manifest early in life it may serve as a marker of increased familial liability to CHD.[1]

LDL receptor activity in cell membranes of normal people is genetically controlled.[1] It has been suggested that a genetically determined low level of receptor activity may be a characteristic of one group of people predisposed to premature CHD.[1]

The anatomical pattern of the coronary tree is probably genetically determined,[78] and the susceptibility of the arterial wall to atherosclerosis may in man, as well as in animals, be genetically determined.[76,78] It has been suggested that not only the extent but also the predilection sites of atherosclerotic lesions could show familial resemblance. Likewise, the hereditary influences on clotting mechanisms may be related to the familial occurrence of CHD.[21] Other risk factors affecting the familial predisposition to the disease remain to be found among the 246 suggested coronary risk factors,[79] or from entirely new sources.

SUMMARY

Coronary heart disease (CHD) aggregates in families. The familial component is most conspicuous in early-onset CHD. Major coronary risk factors also show familial resemblance which results from shared genetic and environmental influences and from their interaction. Nevertheless, the distinct familial components in blood pressure, serum total, low-density lipoprotein (LDL) and high-density lipoprotein (HDL) cholesterol fail to account fully for the familial component in CHD. Other familial risk factors thus remain to be found for much familial CHD.

REFERENCES

[1]Berg K. Genetics of coronary heart disease. Prog Med Genet 1983; 5: 35–90.
[2]Gertler MM, White PD. Coronary heart disease in young adults: a multidisciplinary study. Cambridge, Mass: Harvard University, 1954.

[3]Shanoff HM, Little A, Murphy EA, Rykert HE. Studies of male survivors of myocardial infarction due to 'essential' atherosclerosis. I. Characteristics of the patients. Can Med Assoc J 1961; 84: 519–32.

[4]Rose G. Familial patterns of ischaemic heart disease. Br J Prev Soc Med 1964; 18: 75–80.

[5]Phillips RL, Lilienfeld AM, Diamond EL, Kagan A. Frequency of coronary heart disease and cerebrovascular accidents in parents and sons of coronary heart disease index cases and controls. Am J Epidemiol 1974; 100: 87–100.

[6]Welin L. Family study on ischaemic heart disease and its risk factors. Göteborg, Sweden: University of Göteborg, 1978. (Thesis)

[7]Thordarsson O, Fridriksson S. Aggregation of deaths from ischaemic heart disease among first and second degree relatives of 108 males and 42 females with myocardial infarction. Acta Med Scand 1979; 205: 493–500.

[8]Rissanen AM. Familial occurrence of coronary heart disease and its risk factors. A study on 415 families of young and middle-aged Finnish men with and without coronary heart disease. Helsinki, Finland: University of Helsinki, 1980. (Thesis)

[9]Hamby RI. Hereditary aspects of coronary artery disease. Am Heart J 1981; 101: 639–49.

[10]Rosenberg L, Miller DR, Kaufman DW et al. Myocardial infarction in women under 50 years of age. JAMA 1983; 250: 2801–6.

[11]Rissanen AM, Nikkilä EA. Coronary artery disease and its risk factors in families of young men with angina pectoris and in controls. Br Heart J 1977; 39: 875–83.

[12]Rissanen AM. Familial aggregation of coronary heart disease in a high incidence area (North Karelia, Finland). Br Heart J 1979; 42: 294–303.

[13]Rissanen AM. Familial occurrence of coronary heart disease: effect of age at diagnosis. Am J Cardiol 1979; 44: 60–6.

[14]ten Kate LP, Boman H, Daiger SP, Motulsky AG. Familial aggregation of coronary heart disease and its relation to known genetic risk factors. Am J Cardiol 1982; 50: 945–53.

[15]Rissanen AM, Nikkilä EA. Familial coronary heart disease: identification of the high-risk groups. Atherosclerosis 1984; 53: 27–46.

[16]Slack J, Evans KA. The increased risk of death from ischaemic heart disease in first degree relatives of 121 men and 96 women with ischaemic heart disease. J Med Genet 1966; 3: 239–57.

[17]Forde OH, Thelle DS. The Troms, heart study; risk factors for coronary heart disease related to the occurrence of myocardial infarction in first degree relatives. Am J Epidemiol 1977; 105: 192–9.

[18]Thelle DS, Forde OH. The cardiovascular study in Finnmark County: coronary risk factors and the occurrence of myocardial infarction in first degree relatives and in subjects of different ethnic origin. Am J Epidemiol 1979; 110: 708–15.

[19]Nora JJ, Lortscher RH, Spangler RD, Nora AH, Kimberling WJ. Genetic-epidemiologic study of early-onset ischemic heart disease. Circulation 1980; 61: 503–8.

[20]Epstein FH. Hereditary aspects of coronary heart disease. Am Heart J 1964; 67: 445–56.

[21]Murphy EA. Some difficulties in the investigation of genetic factors in coronary artery disease. Can Med Assoc J 1967; 97: 1181–92.

[22]Sholtz RI, Rosenman RH, Brand RJ. The relationship of reported parental history to the incidence of coronary heart disease in the Western Collaborative Group study. Am J Epidemiol 1975; 102: 350–6.

[23]Hammond EC, Garfinkel L, Seidman H. Longevity of parents and grandparents in relation to heart disease and associated variables. Circulation 1971; 43: 31–44.

[24]Deutscher S, Epstein FH, Kjellsberg MO. Familial aggregation of factors associated with coronary heart disease. Circulation 1966; 33: 911–24.

[25]Deutscher S, Epstein FH, Keller JB. Relationships between familial aggregation of coronary heart disease and risk factors in the general population. Am J Epidemiol 1969; 89: 510–20.

[26]Deutscher S, Ostrander LD, Epstein FH. Familial factors in premature coronary heart disease—a preliminary report from the Tecumseh Community Heart Study. Am J Epidemiol 1970; 91: 233–7.

[27]Snowden CB, McNamara PM, Garrison RJ, Feinleib M, Kannel WB, Epstein FH. Predicting coronary heart disease in siblings—a multivariate assessment. The Framingham heart study. Am J Epidemiol 1982; 115: 217–22.

[28]Williams RR, Skolnick M, Carmelli D et al. Utah pedigree studies: design and preliminary data for premature male CHD deaths. Prog Clin Biol Res 1979; 32: 711–29.

[29]Thomas CB, Cohen BH. Familial occurrence of hypertension and coronary artery disease, with observations concerning obesity and diabetes. Ann Intern Med 1955; 42: 90–127.

[30]Kannel WB. Coronary risk factors, II. Prospects for prevention of atherosclerosis in the young. Aust NZ J Med 1976; 6: 410–9.

[31]Harvald B, Hauge M. Coronary occlusion in twins. Acta Genet Med Gemellol (Roma) 1970; 19: 248–50.

[32]de Faire U. Ischaemic heart disease in death discordant twins. Acta Med Scand 1974; suppl 568.

[33]Dimsdale JE, Gilbert J, Hutter AM, Hackett TP, Block PC. Predicting cardiac morbidity based on risk factors and coronary angiographic findings. Am J Cardiol 1981; 47: 73–6.

[34]Anderson AJ, Loeffler RF, Barboriak JJ, Rimm AA. Occlusive coronary artery disease and parental history of myocardial infarction. Prev Med 1979; 8: 419–28.

[35]Vanhaecke J, Piessens J, Willems JL, De Geest H. Coronary arterial lesions in young men who survived a first myocardial infarction: clinical and electrocardiographic predictors of multivessel disease. Am J Cardiol 1981; 47: 810–4.

[36]Heiberg A, Slack J. Family similarities in the age at coronary death in familial hypercholesterolaemia. Br Med J 1977; 2: 493–5.

[37]Feinleib M, Garrison RJ. The contribution of family studies to the partitioning of population variation of blood pressure. Prog Clin Biol Res 1979; 32: 653–73.

[38]Childs B, Causes of essential hypertension. Prog Med Genet 1983; 5: 1–34.

[39]Williams RR, Hunt SC, Kuida H, Smith JB, Ash KO. Sodium-lithium countertransport in erythrocytes of hypertension prone families in Utah. Am J Epidemiol 1983; 118: 338–44.

[40]Bengtsson C. Ischaemic heart disease in women. Acta Med Scand 1973: suppl 549.

[41]Pagnan A, Donadon W, Ferrai S et al. Study on the risk factors of coronary heart disease in family aggregates of Verona. G Ital Cardiol 1974; 4: 249–60.

[42]Berglund G, Wilhelmsen L. Factors related to blood pressure in a general population sample of Swedish men. Acta Med Scand 1975; 198: 291–8.

[43]Bjartveit K, Foss OP, Gjervik T. The cardiovascular disease study in Norwegian counties. Results from first screening. Acta Med Scand 1983: suppl 675.

[44]Laskarzewski P, Morrison JA, Horvitz R et al. The relationship of parental history of myocardial infarction, hypertension, diabetes and stroke to coronary heart disease risk factors in their adult progeny. Am J Epidemiol 1981; 113: 290–305.

[45]Gudmundsson S, Thorgeirsson G, Thorsteinsson T, Sigfusson N, Sigurdsson G. Risk factor screening amongst first degree relatives of patients with myocardial infarction. Dan Med Bull 1983; 30: 259–62.

[46]Robertson FW. The genetic component in coronary heart disease—a review. Genet Res 1981; 37: 1–16.

[47]Goldstein JL, Brown MS. Familial hypercholesterolemia. In: Stanbury JB, Wyngaarden JB, Fredrickson DS, Goldstein JL, Brown MS, eds. The metabolic basis of inherited disease. 5th ed. New York: Mcgraw-Hill, 1982; 672–712.

[48]Aro A. Serum lipids and lipoproteins in first degree relatives of young survivors of myocardial infarction. Acta Med Scand 1973: suppl 553.

[49]Goldstein JL, Schrott HG, Hazzard WR, Bierman EL, Motulsky AG. Hyperlipidemia in coronary heart disease. II. Genetic analysis of lipid levels in 176 families and delineation of a new inherited disorder, combined hyperlipidemia. J Clin Invest 1973; 52: 1544–68.

[50]Brown MS, Goldstein JL, Fredrickson DS. Familial type 3 hyperlipoproteinemia (Dysbetalipoproteinemia). In: Stanbury JB, Wyngaarden JB, Fredrickson DS, Goldstein JL, Brown MS, eds. The metabolic basis of inherited disease. 5th ed. New York: McGraw-Hill, 1982: 655–71.

[51]Nikkilä EA. Familial lipoprotein lipase deficience and related disorders of chylomicron metabolism. In: Stanbury JB, Wyngaarden JB, Fredrickson DS, Goldstein JL, Brown MS, eds. The metabolic basis of inherited disease. 5th ed. New York: McGraw-Hill, 1982: 622–42.

[52]Brunzell JD, Schrott HG, Motulsky AG, Bierman EL. Myocardial infarction in familial forms of hypertriglyceridemia. Metabolism 1976; 25: 313–20.

[53]Patterson D, Slack J. Lipid abnormalities in male and female survivors of myocardial infarction and their first-degree relatives. Lancet 1972; 1: 393–9.

[54]Schrott HG, Clarke WR, Wiebe DA, Connor WE, Lauer RM. Increased coronary mortality in relatives of hypercholesterolemic school children: the Muscatine Study. Circulation 1979; 59: 320–6.

[55]Ibrahim MA, Pinsky W, Kohn RM, Binette PJ, Winkelstein W. Coronary heart disease: screening by familial aggregation. Pilot study. Arch Environ Health 1968; 16: 235–40.

[56]Moll PP, Sing CF, Weidman WH et al. Total cholesterol and lipoproteins in school children: prediction of coronary heart disease in adult relatives. Circulation 1983; 67: 127–34.

[57]Rissanen AM, Nikkilä EA. Aggregation of coronary risk factors in families of men with fatal and non-fatal coronary heart disease. Br Heart J 1979; 42: 373–80.

[58]Robertson FW, Cumming AM. Genetic and environmental variation in serum lipoproteins in relation to coronary heart disease. J Med Genet 1979; 16: 85–100.

30

[59]Levine RS, Hennekens CH, Rosner B, Gourley J, Gelband H, Jesse MJ. Cardiovascular risk factors among children of men with premature myocardial infarction. Public Health Rep 1981; 96: 60.

[60]Micheli H, Pometta D, Jornot C, Scherrer J-R. High density lipoprotein cholesterol in male relatives of patients with coronary heart disease. Atherosclerosis 1979; 32: 269–76.

[61]Glueck CJ, Fallat RW, Tsang R, Buncher CR. Hyperlipemia in progeny of parents with myocardial infarction before age 50. Am J Dis Child 1974; 127: 70–5.

[62]Schrott HG, Clarke WR, Abrahams P, Wiebe DA, Lauer RM. Coronary artery disease mortality in relatives of hypertriglyceridemic schoolchildren. The muscatine study. Circulation 1982; 65: 300–5.

[63]Glueck CJP, Gartside P, Fallat RW, Sulski J, Steiner PM. Longevity syndromes: familial hypobeta and familial hyperalpha lipoproteinemia. J Lab Clin Med 1976; 88: 941–57.

[64]Nupuf MS, Sutherland WHF. High density lipoprotein levels in children of young men with ischaemic heart disease. Atherosclerosis 1979; 33: 365–70.

[65]Franzen J, Fex G. High density lipoprotein composition versus heredity for acute myocardial infarction in middle-aged males. Acta Med Scand 1982; 211: 121–4.

[66]Köbberling J, Tattersall R. The genetics of diabetes mellitus. London: Academic Press, 1982.

[67]Laskarzewski PM, Khoury P, Morrison JA, Kelly K, Mellies MJ, Glueck CJ. Familial obesity and leanness. Int J Obes 1983; 7: 505–27.

[68]Salber EJ, MacMahon B. Cigarette smoking among high school students related to social class and parental smoking habits. Am J Public Health 1961; 51: 1780–9.

[69]Kaprio J, Koskenvuo M, Sarna S. Cigarette smoking, use of alcohol, and leisure-time physical activity among same sexed adult male twins. In: Twin research III: Epidemiological and clinical studies. New York: Alan R Liss, 1981: 37–46.

[70]Haynes SG, Eaker ED, Feinleib M. Spouse behavior and coronary heart disease in men: prospective results from the Framingham heart study. I. Concordance of risk factors and the relationship of psychosocial status to coronary incidence. Am J Epidemiol 1983; 118: 1–22.

[71]Siegel AJ, Hennekens CH, Rosner B, Karlson LK. Paternal history of coronary heart disease reported by marathon runners. N Engl J Med 1979; 301: 90–1.

[72]Friedman CD, Klatsky AL, Siegelaub AB, McCarthy N. Kaiser-Permanente epidemiologic study of myocardial infarction. Am J Epidemiol 1974; 99: 101–16.

[73]Hedstrand H, Aberg H. Familial history in males at low and high risk for cardiovascular disease. Prev Med 1978; 7: 15–21.

[74]Heller RF, Kelson MC. Family history in 'low risk' men with coronary heart disease. J Epidemiol Community Health 1983; 37: 29–31.

[75]Sigurdsson G, Sigfusson N, Thorsteinsson T, Olafsson O, Davidsson D, Samuelsson S. Screening for health risks. How useful is a questionnaire response showing a positive family history of myocardial infarction, hypertension or cerebral stroke? Acta Med Scand 1983; 213: 45–50.

[76]McGill HC Jr. Atherosclerosis: problems in endpoints for genetic analysis. In: Sing CF, Skolnick M, eds. Genetic analysis of common diseases: Applications to predictive factors in coronary disease. New York: Alan R Liss, 1979: 27–49.

[77]Brunzell JD, Sniderman AD, Albers JJ, Kwiterovich PO. Apoproteins B and A-I and coronary artery disease in humans. Arteriosclerosis 1984; 4: 79–83.

[78]Neufeld HN, Goldbourt U. Coronary heart disease: genetic aspects. Circulation 1983; 67: 943–54.

[79]Hopkins PN, Williams RR. A survey of 246 suggested coronary risk factors. Atherosclerosis 1981; 40: 1–52.

Discussion on Chapter 3

Oliver
You hinted that there might be familial differences, maybe even genetic differences, in the different clinical manifestations of the disease.

Rissanen
There are two studies where this has been examined. First were the family studies on Finnish males with various manifestations of coronary heart disease. The overall rate of coronary heart disease was similar in families of all affected men. However, in families in which the proband had had a fatal myocardial infarction there was an excess of coronary deaths among the relatives, whereas if the proband had angina there was an excess of non-fetal forms of the disease among asymptomatic relatives. Second is the Utah Pedigree study now in progress.

Haynes
It is quite instructive to realise that there may be a large genetic component to the disease among individuals under the age of 50 but less so in the over-50s. Do you agree?

Rissanen
In most populations the familial or genetic component is more conspicuous at an early age, but definite age limits cannot be stated. The expression of a familial component varies, depending mainly on the environment.

Shapiro
Just on that point you seem a little disturbed by the difference in the magnitude of the risk, given a family history, in the case control studies as against the follow-up studies—particularly Framingham. The Framingham study enrolled people at about age 40 and they had to be followed before they got their infarct. The case control studies tended to enrol younger people, so the findings from Framingham and from the studies that you referred to may in fact be entirely compatible.

Haynes
The Framingham study began in 1950 with individuals aged 29–59. They have recently analysed their data in terms of three 8 year follow-up periods. In each of these follow-up periods the strength of the coronary risk factors tends to be the same. This would suggest that whether we are dealing with younger cases or older cases, the measurements made in that study seem to be fairly consistent over time despite the aging of the cohort.

Rissanen
The Framingham population is probably a bit different from most of the Finnish populations I was referring to earlier.

Oliver

I have always assumed that the possible differences in the degree of the penetration of the familial or genetic factor in relation to age is due to dilution. If more people die in the earlier age groups in relation to familial influences, then fewer will be identifiable in the older age groups.

Haynes

When 50% or more of the disease is genetic in nature, we do not know what that actually means for prevention. Does it mean that part of the disease is not preventable?

Rissanen

Familial or genetic liability to coronary heart disease may not be expressed in certain environments, and providing such environments leaves much room for prevention. There are families with clear familial type II hypercholesterolaemia where the previous generation has lived well on into old age despite a clear genetic proneness to coronary heart disease. A totally dominant genetic component is very rare. We have, however, in our studies of young men with coronary heart disease seen it in the few families in which the mother too was affected at an early age. Half of the daughters of such mothers as well as their sons had coronary heart disease at a very early age, independently of the environment.

Slack

The definition of heritability is not that it is the amount of genetic material contributing to coronary artery disease, from which you might conclude that there is little to be done about environment. The definition of heritability is the proportion of genetic contribution to the variance compared with the total variance of liability. It does not mean that there is a single genetic component which is inalterable.

$$\text{Heritability } (h^2) = \frac{\text{Genetic variance in liability}}{\text{Total variance in liability}}$$

If liability to a disorder is normally distributed in a population a small shift of the distribution, whether due to genetic or environmental factors, will cause a surprisingly large difference in incidence in a population.

4. Gonadal hormones, lipoprotein metabolism and coronary heart disease

E.A. Nikkilä, M.J. Tikkanen and T. Kuusi

It is becoming increasingly evident that lipoprotein abnormalities have a key position in the pathogenesis of atherosclerosis and coronary heart disease (CHD). Raised levels of very-low-density (VLDL) or low-density (LDL) lipoproteins or subnormal concentrations of high-density lipoproteins (HDL) are almost a sine qua non for premature development of atherosclerosis, the other risk factors like smoking and hypertension playing only a contributory role. The overall prevalence and incidence of atherosclerotic vascular disease in populations are mainly functions of the average level of LDL, whereas the concentration of HDL may be more important on an individual basis. Nevertheless, the ratio between the concentrations of LDL and HDL or between their major apoproteins, apo B and apo A-I, have appeared to be the best predictors of future coronary events. [1,2]

Early studies on plasma lipoproteins in man established definite sex differences which were compatible with the known higher incidence of atherosclerotic vascular disease in men than in premenopausal women. Thus, women were shown to have higher average levels of HDL lipids but lower concentrations of VLDL than men.[3-5] On the other hand, the LDL levels did not show any major differences between the sexes before middle age. At the same time, it was shown that oestrogenic hormones raised the HDL levels in men[6,7] whereas androgen treatment was followed by a remarkable fall in HDL, often combined with a simultaneous rise in LDL levels.[6-9]

These observations led to some enthusiastic trials which aimed at preventing CHD in men by giving oestrogenic hormones. The possible advantages achieved by changing the lipoprotein pattern were completely masked, however, by the severe side effects of oestrogens and the treatment was soon abandoned. The introduction of oral contraceptive pills then diverted attention to the possible adverse effects of oestrogens on the plasma lipoprotein pattern in women of fertile age. It was shown that the pills containing different combinations of oestrogen and progestational steroids increased plasma triglyceride, VLDL and LDL concentrations with simultaneous suppression of HDL.[10,11] The changes were attributed either to the oestrogen component or to the androgenic activity of many of the synthetic progestagens. Only recently have the lipid metabolic effects of each category of sex steroids been exactly defined. In the course of these studies it has been found that each gonadal hormone influences plasma lipoprotein concentrations by several independent mechanisms and that the effects in premenopausal women may be different from those observed in postmenopausal women and in men.

EFFECTS OF OESTROGENIC HORMONES ON LIPOPROTEINS

Oestrogens influence the metabolism of all three major plasma lipoproteins. In animal experiments pharmacological doses of oestrogens stimulate the hepatic synthesis of VLDL,[12,13] and increase the catabolism of LDL[14] by enhancing the binding and uptake of LDL particles into the liver.[15] In premenopausal women the use of oral contraceptive pills with a high oestrogen content is associated with a pronounced rise in VLDL concentration,[11,16] which is based on increased production of VLDL particles.[7-19] The composition of VLDL is not significantly altered by oestrogens.[20,21] Among postmenopausal women oestrogen substitution does not influence the plasma triglyceride or VLDL levels.[21,22] Even so, in population studies the postmenopausal women using hormones have higher triglyceride and VLDL levels than those without hormones.[23,24] It is likely that the lipoprotein effects depend on the dose and nature of the oestrogen preparation used.

In accordance with the results of animal experiments, oestrogens have been shown to decrease the concentration of LDL in men and in postmenopausal women.[6,22,25,26] This effect is not observed in premenopausal women using oestrogens in combination with progestins as contraceptive pills. In these women the LDL mass concentration measured as Sf 0–12 fraction in ultracentrifuge analysis may even be increased[10,11,16] in spite of unchanged LDL cholesterol levels.[20,21] This apparent discrepancy is explained by the fact that oestrogens change the composition of LDL particles by increasing their triglyceride and phospholipid contents relative to that of cholesterol.[6,20,26,27] Thus, the cholesterol/phospholipid and cholesterol/protein ratios of LDL are reduced by oestrogens, the LDL particles become enriched with triglyceride and their density increases as indicated by a decreasing average flotation rate (Sf value).[11,16] It is not known, however, whether these compositional changes make the LDL particle more or less atherogenic in comparison with the normal female LDL. It is likely that the increased LDL concentration observed in pill users is related to the androgenic or antioestrogenic properties of the progestin component rather than to the oestrogen. In postmenopausal women the extent of the fall in LDL levels by oestrogen is directly proportional to the pretreatment level and thus oestrogens are highly effective in the treatment of postmenopausal hyper-LDL-aemia (type 2 hyper-cholesterolaemia).[22] No reports have been published on the LDL kinetics during oestrogen administration in human beings and it is therefore not clear whether the lowering of plasma LDL concentrations by oestrogenic hormones is based on diminished formation or on accelerated catabolism of LDL particles. The fact that VLDL and apo B production and turnover are increased by oestrogens[28] favours the second alternative and support is also given for this mechanism by the observation in animals that oestrogens increase LDL binding to the liver.[15]

The concentration of HDL is regularly raised by oestrogens in both sexes and at all ages. The effect of contraceptive pills on plasma HDL is dependent on the oestrogen-to-progestin ratio and on the androgenic activity of the latter steroid.[24,29]

Thus, preparations containing a relatively high amount of oestrogen combined with a progestin with low androgenic activity tend to increase the HDL levels while low-oestrogen pills containing a highly androgenic progestin such as levonorgestrel may cause a substantial fall in HDL. Of the HDL subfractions only the HDL_2 class seems to increase during oestrogen treatment while no change can be observed in the concentration of HDL_3 particles.[30-32] This finding agrees with the fact that females have higher HDL_2 than males whereas there is no sex difference in the HDL_3 levels.[33] In analogy with their effect on LDL, the oestrogenic hormones also modify the composition of HDL. The particles are enriched with triglyceride but become relatively depleted of cholesterol.[20,21]

The mechanisms by which oestrogenic hormones raise the HDL_2 levels in plasma are not absolutely clear but there are probably several separate effects. One study on the HDL apoprotein kinetics showed that oestrogen substitution in postmenopausal women increased the apo A-I synthetic rate but did not influence the catabolism of either apo A-I or apo A-II.[28] Oestrogen treatment does not affect the HDL binding to rat liver membranes.[15] A major mediator of the oestrogen effect on HDL_2 is probably hepatic endothelial lipase.[31] This enzyme is present in endothelial cells lining the liver sinusoids and it selectively hydrolyses the HDL_2 triglycerides and phospholipids and is responsible for the partial removal of HDL_2 lipids from the circulation.[34] Oestrogens suppress the activity of this enzyme,[31,35,36] as a result of which hepatic metabolism of HDL_2 decreases leading to an accumulation of HDL_2 particles into plasma.

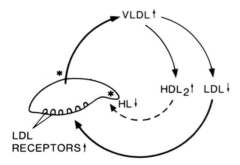

Fig. 4.1 Mode of action of oestrogenic hormones on lipoprotein metabolism. Oestrogens (1) increase the hepatic secretion of VLDL, (2) increase the number of LDL receptors in the liver, and (3) decrease (inhibit?) the activity of hepatic endothelial lipase. As a result of these changes, the VLDL and HDL_2 levels rise whereas the LDL levels decrease.

The various effects of oestrogenic hormones on lipoprotein metabolism are depicted in Figure 4.1.

EFFECTS OF PROGESTATIONAL STEROIDS ON LIPOPROTEIN METABOLISM

The early studies on the role of sex hormones in lipoprotein metabolism did not include progestational hormones. Progesterone itself was found to be relatively indifferent in this respect.[7,37] Even after the introduction of synthetic progesterone analogues as components of oral contraceptives, the lipid effects were attributed mainly to the oestrogen part of the pill. It was soon recognised, however, that progestational steroids are not all similar in their effects on plasma lipids and lipoproteins but that the 19-nortestosterone derivatives, in particular, may be remarkably active on cholesterol, triglyceride and lipoprotein metabolism.[38] Thus, norethindrone acetate given with oestrogen in the pill was shown to abolish all the effects of oestrogen on serum lipids and lipoproteins,[39] to reduce the HDL[10] and raise the LDL levels.[10,11] This compound was also found to decrease the serum triglyceride levels in patients with severe (type 5) hypertriglyceridaemia so that it was even recommended as an effective drug for treatment of this condition.[40]

It is now well recognised that the activity of different progestational steroids on plasma lipoproteins is mainly related to their androgenic or antioestrogenic potency. When used in combination with oestrogens, as is often the case, the net effect depends on the nature of the progestin and on the oestrogen/progestin dose ratio.[29,41] During recent years much attention has been focused on the anticipated adverse effects of progestins on HDL. On the basis of one study[42] it has been assumed that lowering HDL, and particularly HDL_2, concentrations by androgenic progestins increases the risk of atherosclerotic vascular disease. This has led to the development of new progesterone analogues with less androgenic activity.

Triglycerides and VLDL

Progestational steroids with low androgenic activity do not appreciably influence plasma triglyceride or VLDL levels.[37,43,44] They may, however, abolish the oestrogen-induced increases in VLDL production and serum triglyceride concentrations[45] and enhance the plasma clearance of endogenous and exogenous triglycerides.[46] A significant lowering of plasma VLDL triglyceride has recently been observed during treatment with a weakly androgenic progestin, desogestrel.[47]

The nortestosterone-derived progestins (norethindrone, levonorgestrel) tend to reduce the serum triglyceride levels when given either alone[40,48-50] or in combination with low-dose oestrogens.[41,51] In postmenopausal women a combination of levonorgestrel and oestrogen substitution results in a significant lowering of total triglyceride and VLDL levels.[52]

The decrease in VLDL concentrations by progestin treatment is apparently based both on diminished production and accelerated removal of VLDL particles. Norethindrone acetate has been shown to inhibit splanchnic triglyceride secretion in swine[53] and to diminish the release of triglycerides from isolated rat hepatocytes.[54] The clearance of triglycerides from the plasma is increased by progestins.[46,55] The women using combined oral contraceptive pills also show an increased triglyceride-removal efficiency which has been attributed to the progestin component.[17]

LDL

In most studies the different progestational steroids have been without significant effect on plasma LDL cholesterol levels. Slight increases in LDL cholesterol and LDL triglyceride levels have been noted in users of oral contraceptives containing the highly androgenic levonorgestrel.[24,56] Nevertheless, the rise in LDL triglyceride may be attributed to the oestrogen components which the progestin fails to antagonise as efficiently as the increase in VLDL.

HDL

The progestins reduce the plasma HDL levels in a dose-dependent manner. The effect is relatively weak with less androgenic compounds such as progesterone,[7,57] medroxyprogesterone acetate[44,52,58] and desogestrel,[47,59] but becomes quite remarkable when strongly androgenic progestins such as norethindrone[44,50,58] and norgestrel are used.[44,52,58] The latter steroids completely offset the HDL-increasing effect of oestrogens[29,60] the net change of HDL being closely related to the dose ratio of oestrogen vs progestin.[41] In addition, the plasma apo A-I levels are reduced by norgestrel[61] and the HDL cholesterol and phospholipids decrease to about the same extent.[44] Of the two HDL subfractions, the HDL_2 is reduced more than HDL_3[30,31,50,52,57,60,62] which may remain unaffected.[31,52,60,62]

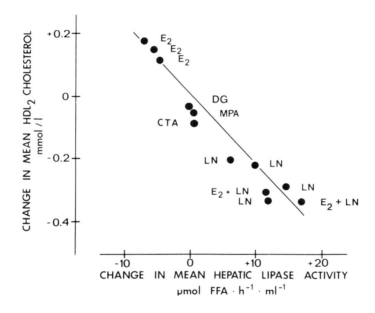

Fig. 4.2 A summary plot on changes produced by different sex steroids in HDL_2 cholesterol vs postheparin plasma hepatic lipase activity. Mean values taken from references 31, 47, 52, 60 and 62. E_2 = oestradiol, DG = desogestrel, MPA = medroxyprogesterone acetate, CTA = cyproterone acetate, LN = levonorgestrel.

The mode of action of progestational steroids on HDL is not completely understood but seems to be mediated, at least partly, by hepatic endothelial lipase. The progestins increase the hepatic lipase activity and reverse the oestrogen-induced suppression of this enzyme.[52,60,62] The magnitude of the effect on HDL and HDL_2 (decrease) by the different progestins parallels the increase in hepatic lipase activity induced by these compounds[63,64] (Fig. 4.2). Thus, medroxyprogesterone[52] and desogestrel[47] are virtually without effect on hepatic lipase while levonorgestrel

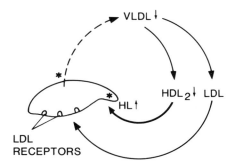

Fig. 4.3 Mode of action of androgenic hormones (androgens, some progestins and anabolic steroids) on lipoprotein metabolism. These hormones (1) decrease the hepatic secretion of VLDL and (2) act as a powerful inducer of hepatic endothelial lipase. These changes are reflected as a decreased concentration of VLDL and as a fall in HDL_2.

causes a remarkable increase in postheparin plasma hepatic lipase activity within 2 weeks.[52,62] It is possible that the inhibition of the hepatic VLDL secretion by progestins (see above) contributes to the decrease in HDL_2 by reducing the mass of VLDL surface components transferred to HDL.

The effects of progestins on plasma lipoprotein metabolism are summarised in Figure 4.3.

EFFECTS OF ANDROGENIC AND ANABOLIC HORMONES ON LIPOPROTEIN METABOLISM

Giving exogenous androgenic hormones such as methyltestosterone to men is followed by a reduction in HDL[26,27,65] and VLDL[26,27] levels. Similar changes are produced by anabolic steroids,[66,67] which may also increase the LDL concentration.[66,68] The reduction in triglyceride and VLDL levels by androgenic steroids is particularly prominent in subjects with hypertriglyceridaemia.[27] The effect is based on decreased production of VLDL but there is also evidence of an acceleration of triglyceride clearance during treatment with anabolic steroids.[46,66]

It is likely that all steroids with androgenic activity selectively reduce the HDL_2 subfraction concentration but leave HDL_3 relatively intact. This has been well documented in the case of anabolic steroids (oxandrolone, stanozolol), which may cause a dramatic fall or even disappearance of HDL_2 particles with only a slight decrease in HDL_3.[68,69] In accordance with this, the apo A-I levels are reduced more than those of apo A-II.[68,70] All these steroids are also powerful inducers of hepatic endothelial lipase[35,68,71] and it is therefore highly plausible that the fall in HDL_2 should be mediated by the increased activity of hepatic lipase. Both effects can be elicited already by very small doses of anabolic steroids and the dose-response curves of HDL_2 and hepatic lipase will parallel each other.[72] Even so, both testosterone[73] and anabolic steroids[70] also suppress the synthesis of apo A-I and this may contribute to the androgen-induced lowering of HDL by a mechanism independent on the hepatic lipase induction.

IMPLICATIONS TO ATHEROSCLEROSIS AND CHD

The effect of sex on the risk of atherosclerotic vascular disease is well explained by the sex differences in plasma lipoprotein concentrations. It is not known, however, whether the lower VLDL and higher HDL and HDL_2 concentrations observed in women really account for the lesser degree of atherosclerosis in women than in men. The changes produced in plasma total HDL and HDL_2 concentrations by exogenous gonadal hormones correspond to the sex difference present in HDL, but the effects on VLDL do not account for the higher VLDL in men compared to females. The relationship between plasma levels of endogenous sex hormones and HDL is completely the opposite of what one might expect, however, and men surviving a myocardial infarction show increased plasma oestrogen levels but have subnormal HDL concentrations.[74] Moreover, plasma testosterone levels are positively and not inversely correlated with HDL cholesterol.[75,76] The development of postmenopausal oestrogen deficiency is not associated with any decrease in plasma HDL levels. These discrepancies are still not explained but they indicate that the relationships between sex hormone status, lipoproteins and atherosclerosis are probably not as straightforward as they have seemed in the past.

Another open question relates to the association between HDL and atherosclerosis. The decrease in HDL (HDL_2) that follows an androgen-induced increase in hepatic lipase activity is thought to be caused by an accelerated hepatic uptake of lipids from HDL_2 particles. This raises the possibility that an increased rate of flux of HDL particles through the plasma promotes the reverse cholesterol transport and inhibits atherogenesis in spite of the fact that the actual concentration of HDL particles is reduced. If this is the case, the subjects with low HDL should be divided into two categories, one with a low and the other with a high turnover rate of HDL particles (not necessarily reflected as low or high turnover rates of apo A-I). Of these two metabolic states the first is probably more atherogenic.

ACKNOWLEDGMENT

Supported by grants from Finnish State Medical Research Council and from Sigrid Jusélius Foundation.

REFERENCES

[1] Brunzell JD, Sniderman AD, Albers JJ, Kwiterovich PO Jr. Apoproteins B and A-I and coronary artery disease in humans. Arteriosclerosis 1984; 4: 79–83.

[2] Castelli W. Epidemiology of coronary heart disease: the Framingham study. Am J Med 1984; 76(2A): 4–12.

[3] Gofman JW, Jones HB, Lindgren FT, Lyon TP, Elliot HA, Strisower B. Blood lipids and human atherosclerosis. Circulation 1950; 2: 161–78.

[4] Russ EM, Eder HA, Barr DP. Protein-lipid relationships in human plasma. I; in normal individuals. Am J Med 1951; 11: 468–79.

[5] Nikkilä E. Studies on lipid-protein relationships in normal and pathological sera and effect of heparin on serum lipoproteins. Scand J Clin Lab Invest 1953; 5(suppl 8): 1–101.

[6] Russ EM, Eder HA, Barr DP. Influence of gonadal hormones on protein-lipid relationships in human plasma. Am J Med 1955; 19: 4–24.

[7]Oliver MF, Boyd GS. The influence of the sex hormones on the circulating lipids and lipoproteins in coronary sclerosis. Circulation 1956; 13: 82–91.

[8]Cramér K. Serum β-lipoprotein lipids and protein during combined administration of dioxydiethylstilbestrol and methyl testosterone. Acta Med Scand 1962; 171: 429–34.

[9]Robinson RW, LeBeau RJ, Cohen WD. Effects of methyl testosterone upon serum lipids. J Clin Endocrinol 1964; 24: 708–13.

[10]Aurell M, Cramér K, Rybo G. Serum lipids and lipoproteins during long-term administration of an oral contraceptive. Lancet 1966; 1: 291–3.

[11]Wynn V, Doar JWH, Mills GL. Some effects of oral contraceptives on serum-lipid and lipoprotein levels. Lancet 1966; 2: 720–3.

[12]Luskey KL, Brown MS, Goldstein JL. Stimulation of the synthesis of very low density lipoproteins in rooster liver by estradiol. J Biol Chem 1974; 249: 5939–47.

[13]Chan L, Jackson RL, O'Malley BW, Means AR. Synthesis of very low density lipoproteins in the cockerel. Effects of estrogen. J Clin Invest 1976; 58: 368–79.

[14]Hay RV, Pottenger LA, Reingold AL, Getz GS, Wissler RW. Degradation of I[125]-labelled serum low density lipoprotein in normal and estrogen-treated male rats. Biochem Biophys Res Comm 1971; 44: 1471–7.

[15]Kovanen PT, Brown MS, Goldstein JL. Increased binding of low density lipoprotein to liver membranes from rats treated with 17 α-ethinyl estradiol. J Biol Chem 1979; 254: 11367–73.

[16]Wynn V, Doar JWH, Mills GL, Stokes T. Fasting serum triglyceride, cholesterol, and lipoprotein levels during oral-contraceptive therapy. Lancet 1969; 2: 756–60.

[17]Kekki M, Nikkilä EA. Plasma triglyceride turnover during use of oral contraceptives. Metabolism 1971; 20: 878–89.

[18]Kissebah AH, Harrigan P, Wynn V. Mechanism of hypertriglyceridaemia associated with contraceptive steroids. Horm Metab Res 1973; 5: 184–90.

[19]Glueck CJ, Fallat RW, Scheel D. Effects of estrogenic compounds on triglyceride kinetics. Metabolism 1975; 24: 537–45.

[20]Rössner S, Larsson-Cohn U, Carlson LA, Boberg J. Effects of an oral contraceptive agent on plasma lipids, plasma lipoproteins, the intravenous fat tolerance and the post-heparin lipoprotein lipase activity. Acta Med Scand 1971; 190: 301–5.

[21]Knopp RH, Walden CE, Wahl PW et al. Oral contraceptive and postmenopausal estrogen effects on lipoprotein triglyceride and cholesterol in an adult female population: relationships to estrogen and progestin potency. J Clin Endocrinol Metab 1981; 53: 1123–32.

[22]Tikkanen MJ, Nikkilä EA, Vartiainen E. Natural oestrogen as an effective treatment for type-II hyperlipoproteinaemia in postmenopausal women. Lancet 1978; 2: 490–1.

[23]Heiss G, Tamir I, David CE et al. Lipoprotein-cholesterol distributions in selected North American populations: The Lipid Research Clinics program prevalence study. Circulation 1980; 61: 302–15.

[24]Wahl P, Walden C, Knopp R et al. Effect of estrogen/progestin potency on lipid/lipoprotein cholesterol. N Engl J Med 1983; 308: 862–7.

[25]Barr DP. Some chemical factors in pathogenesis of atherosclerosis. Circulation 1953; 8: 641–54.

[26]Furman RH, Howard RP, Norcia LN, Keaty EC. The influence of androgens, estrogens and related steroids on serum lipids and lipoproteins. Observations in hypogonadal and normal human subjects. Am J Med 1958; 24: 80–97.

[27]Furman RH, Alaupovic P, Howard RP. Effects of androgens and estrogens on serum lipids and the composition and concentration of serum lipoproteins in normolipemic and hyperlipidemic states. Progr Biochem Pharmacol 1967; 2: 215–49.

[28]Schaefer EJ, Foster DM, Zech LA, Lindgren FT, Brewer HB Jr, Levy RI. The effects of estrogen administration on plasma lipoprotein metabolism in premenopausal females. J Clin Endocrinol Metab 1983; 57: 262–7.

[29]Bradley DD, Wingerd J, Petitti DB, Krauss RM, Ramcharan S. Serum high-density-lipoprotein cholesterol in women using oral contraceptives, estrogens and progestins. N Engl J Med 1978; 299: 17–20.

[30]Krauss RM, Lindgren FT, Wingerd J, Bradley DD, Ramcharan S. Effects of estrogens and progestins on high density lipoproteins. Lipids 1979; 14: 113–8.

[31]Tikkanen MJ, Nikkilä EA, Kuusi T, Sipinen S. Effects of oestradiol and levonorgestrel on lipoprotein lipids and postheparin plasma lipase activities in normolipoproteinaemic women. Acta Endocrinol 1982; 99: 630–5.

[32]Cauley JA, LaPorte RE, Kuller LH, Bates M, Sandler RB. Menopausal estrogen use, high density lipoprotein cholesterol subfractions and liver function. Atherosclerosis 1983; 49: 31–9.

[33]Cheung MC, Albers JJ. The measurement of apolipoprotein A-I and A-II levels in men and women by immunoassay. J Clin Invest 1977; 60: 43–50.

[34]Nikkilä EA, Kuusi T, Taskinen M-R. Role of lipoprotein lipase and hepatic endothelial lipase in the metabolism of high density lipoproteins: A novel concept on cholesterol transport in HDL cycle. In: Carlson LA, Pernow B, eds. Metabolic risk factors in ishemic cardiovascular disease. New York: Raven Press, 1982: 205–15.

[35]Glueck CJ, Gartside P, Fallat RW, Mendoza S. Effect of sex hormones on protamine inactivated nd resistant postheparin plasma lipases. Metabolism 1976; 25: 625–32.

[36]Applebaum DM, Goldberg AP, Pykälisto OJ, Brunzell JD, Bazzard WR. Effect of estrogen on post-heparin lipolytic activity. Selective decline in hepatic triglyceride lipase. J Clin Invest 1977; 59: 601–8.

[37]Svanborg A, Vikrot O. The effect of estradiol and progesterone on plasma lipids in oophorectomized women. Acta Med Scand 1966; 179: 615–22.

[38]Furman RH. Gonadal steroid effects on serum lipids. In: Salhnick HA, Kipnis DM, Vande Wiele RL, eds. Metabolic effects of gonadal hormones and contraceptive steroids. New York, London: Plenum Press, 1969: 247–64.

[39]Gustafson A, Svanborg A. Gonadal steroid effects on plasma lipoproteins and individual phospholipids. J Clin Endocrinol Metab 1972; 35: 203–7.

[40]Glueck CJ, Levy RI, Fredrickson DS. Norethindrone acetate, postheparin lipolytic activity, and plasma triglycerides in familial types I, III, IV, and V hyperlipoproteinemia. Studies in 26 patients and 5 normal persons. Ann Intern Med 1971; 75: 345–52.

[41]Larsson-Cohn U, Fånhraeus L, Wallentin L, Zador G. Lipoprotein changes may be minimized by proper composition of a combined oral contraceptive. Fertil Steril 1981; 35: 172–9.

[42]Meade TW, Greenberg G, Thompson SG. Progestogens and cardiovascular reactions associated with oral contraceptives and a comparison of the safety of 50- and 30-μg oestrogen preparations. Br Med J 1980; 280: 1157–61.

[43]Beck P. Effect of progestins on glucose and lipid metabolism. Ann NY Acad Sci 1977; 286: 434–45.

[44]Silfverstolpe G, Gustafson A, Samsioe G, Svanborg A. Lipid metabolic studies in oophorectomized women. Effects of three different progestogens. Acta Obstet Gynecol Scand 1979; suppl 88: 89–95.

[45]Kenagy R, Weinstein I, Heimberg M. The effects of 17 beta-estradiol and progesterone on the metabolism of free fatty acid by perfused livers from normal female and ovariectomized rats. Endocrinology 1981; 108: 1613–21.

[46]Kissebah AH, Harrigan P, Adams PW, Wynn V. Effect of methandienone on free fatty acid and triglyceride turnover in normal females. Horm Metab Res 1973; 5: 275–9.

[47]Kuusi T, Nikkilä EA, Tikkanen MJ, Sipinen S. Effects of two progestins with different androgenic properties on hepatic endothelial lipase and high density lipoprotein$_2$. Atherosclerosis 1985; 54: 251–62.

[48]Brody S, Kerstell J, Nilsson L, Svanborg A. The effects of some ovulation inhibitors on the different plasma lipid fractions. Acta Med Scand 1968; 183: 1–7.

[49]Gowland E, Jones RA. The effect of oral norethisterone on serum lipid levels in premenopausal women. Br J Obstet Gynaecol 1973; 80: 357–9.

[50]Farish E, Fletcher CD, Hart DM, Kitchener H, Sharpe GLM. A long-term study of the effects of norethisterone on lipoprotein metabolism in menopausal women. Clin Chim Acta 1983; 132:193–8.

[51]Larsson-Cohn U, Wallentin L, Zador G. Plasma lipids and high density lipoproteins during oral contraception with different combinations of ethinyl estradiol and levonorgestrel. Horm Metab Res 1979; 11: 437–40.

[52]Tikkanen MJ, Nikkilä EA, Kuusi T, Sipinen S. Different effects of two progestins on plasma high density lipoproteins (HDL$_2$) and postheparin plasma hepatic lipase activity. Atherosclerosis 1981; 40: 365–9.

[53]Wolfe BM, Grac DM. Norethindrone acetate inhibition of splanchnic triglyceride secretion in conscious glucose-fed swine. J Lipid Res 1979; 20: 175–82.

[54]Cheng DCH, Wolfe BM, Norethindrone acetate inhibition of triglyceride synthesis and release by rat hepatocytes. Atherosclerosis 1983; 46: 41–8.

[55]Glueck CJ, Scheel D, Fishback J, Steiner P. Progestagens, anabolic-androgenic compounds, estrogens: effects on triglycerides and postheparin lipolytic enzymes. Lipids 1972; 7: 110–3.

[56]Silfverstolpe G, Gustafson A, Samsioe G, Svanborg A. Lipid and carbohydrate metabolism studies in oophorectomized women: effects produced by the addition of norethisterone acetate to two estrogen preparations. Arch Gynecol 1982; 231: 279–87.

[57]Fånhraeus L, Larsson-Cohn U, Wallentin L. L-norgestrel and progesterone have different influences on plasma lipoproteins. Eur J Clin Invest 1983; 13: 447–53.

[58]Hirvonen E, Mälkönen M, Manninen V. Effects of different progestogens on lipoproteins during postmenopausal replacement therapy. N Engl J Med 1981; 304: 560–3.

[59]Samsioe G. Comparative effects of the oral contraceptive combinations 0.150 mg desogestrel + 0.030 mg ethinyloestradiol and 0.150 mg levonorgestrel + 0.030 mg ethinyloestradiol on lipid and lipoprotein metabolism in healthy female volunteers. Contraception 1982; 25: 487–503.

[60]Tikkanen MJ, Nikkilä EA, Kuusi T, Sipinen S. Effects of oestradiol and levonorgestrel on lipoprotein lipids and postheparin plasma lipase activities in normolipoproteinaemic women. Acta Endocrinol 1982; 99: 630–5.

[61]Havekes L, Van Gent CM, Stegerhoek CI, Arntzenius AC, Hessel LW. High density lipoprotein cholesterol and apolipoprotein A-I levels in 32–33 year-old women on steroid contraceptives— differences between two frequently used low-estrogen pills. Clin Chim Acta 1981; 116: 223–9.

[62]Tikkanen MJ, Nikkilä EA, Kuusi T, Sipinen S. Reduction of plasma high-density lipoprotein$_2$ cholesterol and increase of postheparin plasma hepatic lipase activity during progestin treatment. Clin Chim Acta 1981; 115: 63–71.

[63]Nikkilä EA, Tikkanen MJ, Kuusi T. Effects of progestins on plasma lipoproteins and heparin-releasable lipases. In: Bardin CW, Milgrom E, Mauvais-Jarvis P, eds. Progesterone and progestins. New York: Raven Press, 1983: 415–24.

[64]Kuusi T, Nikkilä EA, Tikkanen MJ, Taskinen M-R, Ehnholm C. Function of hepatic endothelial lipase in lipoprotein metabolism. In: Schettler FG, Gotto AM, Middelhoff G, Habenicht AJR, Jurutka KR, eds. Atherosclerosis VI. New York, Heidelberg, Berlin: Springer, 1983: 628–32.

[65]Barr DP. Influence of sex and sex hormones upon the development of atherosclerosis and upon the lipoproteins of plasma. J Chronic Dis 1955; 1: 63–85.

[66]Olsson AG, Orö L, Rössner S. Effects of oxandrolone on plasma lipoproteins and the intravenous fat tolerance in man. Atherosclerosis 1974; 19: 337–46.

[67]Tamai T, Nakai T, Yamada S et al. Effects of oxandrolone on plasma lipoproteins in patients with type IIa, IIb and IV hyperlipoproteinemia: occurrence of hypo-high density lipoproteinemia. Artery 1979; 5: 125–43.

[68]Taggart HM, Applebaum-Bowden D, Haffner S et al. Reduction in high density lipoproteins by anabolic steroid (Stanozolol) therapy for postmenopausal osteoporosis. Metabolism 1982; 31: 1147–52.

[69]Hara T, Miller JP, Gotto AM Jr, Patsch JR. Oxandrolone and plasma triglyceride reduction: Effect on triglyceride-rich and high density lipoproteins. Artery 1981; 9: 328–41.7

[70]Haffner SM, Kushwaha RS, Foster DM, Applebaum-Bowden D, Hazzard W R. Studies on the metabolic mechanism of reduced high density lipoproteins during anabolic steroid therapy. Metabolism 1983; 32: 413–20.

[71]Ehnholm C, Huttunen JK, Kinnunen PJ, Miettinen TA, Nikkilä EA. Effect of oxandrolone treatment on the activity of lipoprotein lipase, hepatic lipase and phospholipase A, of human postheparin plasma. N Engl J Med 1975; 292: 1314–7.

[72]Nikkilä EA, Kuusi T, Taskinen M-R, Tikkanen MJ. Regulation of lipoprotein metabolism by endothelial lipolytic ensymes. In: Carlson LA, Olsson AG, eds. Treatment of hyperlipoproteinemia. New York: Raven Press, 1984: 77–84.

[73]Solyom A, Bradford RH, Furman RH. Methyltestosterone effect on apolipoprotein A and albumin metabolism in canine serum. Am J Physiol 1971; 221: 1587–95.

[74]Phillips GB, Castelli WP, Abbott RD, McNamara PM. Association of hyperestrogenemia and coronary heart disease in men in the Framingham cohort: Am J Med 1983; 74: 863–9.

[75]Nordoy A, Aakvaag A, Thelle D. Sex hormones and high density lipoproteins in healthy males. Atherosclerosis 1979; 34: 431–6.

[76]Gutai J, LaPorte R, Kuller L, Dai W, Falvo-Gerard L, Caggiula A. Plasma testosterone, high density lipoprotein cholesterol and other lipoprotein fractions. Am J Cardiol 1981; 48: 897–902.

Discussion on Chapter 4

Oliver
Is the apparent male/female difference in lipoprotein lipase response—in relation to free fatty acid release in adipose tissue—true of both heparin and catecholamine-induced lipoprotein lipase activity?

Nikkilä
It is heparin-released lipoprotein lipase. The hormone-sensitive lipase is a different enzyme and has nothing to do with lipoprotein metabolism. There is no sex difference in the activity of hormone-sensitive lipase. The two enzymes are not related to each other.

Beaumont J.-L.
Did you find a difference between women on oral contraception or treated by synthetic sex hormones with and without a thrombosis?

Nikkilä
We did not see any case of thrombosis in our series of pre- or postmenopausal women.

Wynn
Firstly, would you like to comment on the studies done by Glueck and his group on HDL_2 and HDL_3 turnover on the anabolic steroid stanozolol? That study would not exactly confirm your predictions in relation to HDL_2 turnover.

Secondly, what would be the theoretical effect on the atherogenic risk of lowering HDL_2 levels using either anabolic steroids or synthetic progestagens? Theoretically you could argue from your data that lowering HDL_2 levels with an androgen and speeding up the cholesterol transport to the liver and the excretion of cholesterol could possibly be protective—whereas HDL_2 levels relate to the periphery and lowering them could be the reverse of protective, in fact atherogenic. So, is there a contradiction in that situation?

Nikkilä
That is true. We do not know if there could be two types of low HDL. In one case there would be low production of HDL while in other the HDL would decrease due to overutilisation with a rapid turnover. A low HDL due to a high turnover rate, high recycling rate of HDL lipids, might be a good thing in spite of the low HDL level.

Oliver
Have labelled studies not been done?

Nikkilä
Studies with labelled HDL are extremely difficult and would give you only the turnover of the apoprotein moiety. The kinetics of the HDL cholesterol or phospholipids are different from true natural HDL metabolism. In the HDL

particles the apoproteins and labelled cholesterol are exchanged without transfer of mass. The turnover of HDL cholesterol is much more rapid than the turnover of the apoproteins.

Wynn

Perhaps it is overstating the case to argue, as you have done that because the HDL_2 levels are reduced by the use of certain type of progestins and anabolic steroids it follows that the turnover rate of the HDL_2 has also increased.

Nikkilä

The turnover rate of HDL cholesterol and HDL phospholipids is increased but it does not necessarily mean that the overall rate of apo A-I is also increased. The protein may well remain in the particle when the hepatic lipase removes some of the surface phospholipids.

Wynn

But have you really got direct evidence of an increased excretion of cholesterol via the HDL_2 mechanism in a situation of this kind? Is it not really speculation?

Nikkilä

It is speculation, because the measurement of the turnover of HDL components other than just the protein is almost impossible.

Rifkind

Given the current trend to use combined oestrogen and progestin in postmenopausal women on account of endometrial cancer, and concerns that the use of progestins could increase coronary heart disease through the effects on lipoproteins, what combination would you recommend at this time?

Nikkilä

We do not have a good answer. We have progestins which are indifferent regarding lipoprotein metabolism—for example, medroxyprogesterone and desogestrel. My recommendation would be a combination of oestrogenic hormones with this type of progestin.

Oliver

Is it not the case that there is quite a difference in the endometrial cancer rate when comparing premarin with cyclic cycloprogynova, the former being the worse? There is quite an extensive report on this from the Oxford group.

Wynn

To answer your question: the patient being, of course, a woman you have the opportunity of using pretty minimal amounts of progestin for only 5 days in a 21 day cycle—5 or 6 days would be quite enough. All you have to do is to produce menstrual bleeding; you do not actually have to suppress the oestrogen effect on the endometrium permanently. It is shedding the endometrium that counts.

5. Diabetes as a risk factor for coronary heart disease

A. Reunanen

Diabetes is an established risk factor for the three major atherosclerotic complications,[1] of which coronary heart disease (CHD) is the most important from a public health point of view. The association between diabetes and CHD has been extensively described in some recent reviews.[1,2] Diabetes appears to be one of the few coronary risk factors which has a stronger, or at least similar, predictive value in women than in men. Therefore in a symposium like this, which is aimed at showing the special features of CHD in women, it is appropriate to discuss the matter in more detail.

EPIDEMIOLOGY OF DIABETES

Diabetes, which may be defined either as an absolute or as a relative deficiency of insulin, is not a uniform disease but is probably a group of separate diseases having different pathogenesis but presenting with more or less similar findings. Generally, diabetics can be divided into insulin-dependent, or type 1, diabetics and non-insulin-dependent, or type 2, diabetics. The definitions and diagnostic criteria of diabetes have recently been revised.[3,4] In the studies concerning the predictive value of diabetes as a CHD risk factor it is important to take into account the overall and sex-specific prevalence of the disease. The prevalence of type 1 disease does not show a marked age-dependence after puberty being in most Western countries around 0.2–0.4%. There are generally very small differences by sex but in many epidemiological studies the rates have been somewhat greater in men than in women.[2,5] Type 2 diabetes is much more common and there is very marked age-dependence, the rates increasing steeply after 40 years. Because of the prominent age-dependence the prevalence rates depend heavily on the age range and age structure of the population. The overall prevalence of type 2 diabetes in most Western countries is about 2–3%. Type 2 diabetes seems to be more common in men according to many studies in the United States[6,7] but in Finland, for example, type 2 is clearly more common in women.[8]

CORONARY ATHEROSCLEROSIS AND PREVALENCE OF CHD

According to many autopsy and clinical studies[9] the extent of atherosclerotic lesions and clinical myocardial infarction are more common in diabetics than in non-diabetics. In these earlier studies it was also noted that there was hardly any difference between the sexes as far as CHD in diabetics was concerned. In many of these studies patients were selected and little attention was paid to age adjustment. Large international projects confirmed, however, that age-specific prevalence of severe atherosclerosis in coronary arteries was unequivocally higher in diabetics.[10,11] The prevalence of clinical CHD in diabetics and non-diabetics has been investigated to a limited extent. In a recent large multinational study the prevalence of angina and ECG abnormalities were investigated in 14 middle-aged population groups of diabetics.[12] There were considerable differences in prevalence rates between the groups, reflecting mainly the extent of macrovascular complications in the populations from which diabetics were drawn. The prevalence of angina pectoris as well as ECG abnormalities were almost similar in male and female diabetics. Unfortunately, there was no opportunity to study non-diabetic control groups. In a recent Finnish survey the prevalence of CHD was significantly higher in middle-aged newly diagnosed diabetics than in age-matched non-diabetics.[13] In that study, the prevalence of verified myocardial infarction in diabetic women was about the same as in non-diabetic men whereas the prevalence of chest pain symptoms and ECG abnormalities was equally high in both women and men diabetics and much higher than in non-diabetics.

INCIDENCE OF CHD AND PROGNOSIS

Prospective studies in clinical series of diabetics and in unselected populations have given more reliable and more detailed information on the susceptibility of diabetics for CHD. According to the extensive prospective studies carried out on diabetics treated at Joslin's clinic it was evident that female diabetics, almost irrespective of age and duration of the disease, have the same incidence of myocardial infarction as male diabetics of the same age.[14]

The Framingham study was one of the first studies in which the incidence of CHD in diabetics and non-diabetics in unselected populations would be compared.[6] According to the results, CHD mortality risks were higher in female than in male diabetics compared with non-diabetics.[6,15] The high CHD mortality risks of women with diabetes were later confirmed in the Evans County, Bedford and Rancho Bernardo studies.[16-18] To illustrate in more detail CHD mortality risks of men and women with diabetes preliminary results from a large Finnish prospective study are given below.

The study population consisted of 12 572 men and 12 300 women aged 40–69 years drawn from over 30 geographical areas from all parts of the country. 273 of the men and 292 of the women had a history of known diabetes or new diabetes was detected at the baseline investigation. In a mean follow-up time of 10 years 2485 men and 2240 women had died. In 1082 of the deceased men and in 334 of the women the principal cause of death was CHD. The unadjusted CHD death rates for diabetics and non-diabetics are presented in Table 5.1. As expected, CHD mortality was substantially increased in both men and women diabetics. In our study, Finnish female diabetics had more or less the same CHD mortality as non-diabetic men.

This differs from the results obtained in some earlier population studies which found that men and women with diabetes had nearly equal CHD mortality.[15,18] The small number of the deceased women even in such a large study as ours, and the particularly great difference in CHD mortality of men and women in Finland may have contributed to the results.

Table 5.1 CHD mortality (%) in diabetics and non-diabetics aged 40–69 years in a mean follow-up time of 10 years. Number of deceased in parentheses.

| | Age groups (years) | | | |
	40–49	50–59	60–69	All
Men				
Diabetics	18.2	22.4	26.6	23.1
(n=273)	(12)	(22)	(29)	(63)
Non-diabetics	3.6	9.6	17.0	8.3
(n=12 299)	(207)	(396)	(416)	(1019)
Women				
Diabetics	3.2	9.6	16.9	12.0
(n=292)	(1)	(6)	(28)	(35)
Non-diabetics	0.4	2.4	6.4	2.5
(n=12 008)	(22)	(96)	(18)	(299)

There are some peculiar features of myocardial infarction in diabetics. In clinical studies diabetic women with acute myocardial infarction had generally had worse prognosis than diabetic men.[1,19] The mortality excess seemed to be apparent in the acute phase as well as in the immediate postinfarction period. In addition, it has been shown that clinically silent myocardial infarction may be more common in diabetics.[1] This finding can, however, be partly explained by the more thorough and frequent investigations of diabetics.

In the incidence studies dealing with a large number of diabetics the increased CHD morbidity and mortality risk of females applies both to type 1 and type 2 disease. The relative risk of type 1 diabetics has, however, been uniformly greater and manifested at a younger age.[14,20] In population studies the relatively small number of diabetics and lack of relevant baseline data have unfortunately not allowed a detailed investigation of the prognosis by the type of the disease. Even so, in the Framingham study it was clear that those with the greatest cardiovascular mortality risk were female diabetics on insulin therapy. Similar findings have been obtained in our prospective study.

INDEPENDENCE OF DIABETES AS A RISK FACTOR

Diabetes is associated with many factors which affect CHD morbidity and mortality rates. Age is one of the main factors. The highest age-specific CHD mortality risks of diabetics have been observed in younger age groups and the risks decrease gradually with age. In most studies diabetics have excess CHD mortality even at an advanced age but in some studies the excess risk is not more significant in the elderly.[21] In our prospective study the relative risk of diabetics dying from CHD decreased substantially after adjusting for age (Table 5.2). In a more detailed

Table 5.2 Unadjusted relative risks of diabetics dying from CHD and relative risks after adjustment for age and other risk factors.

| | Relative risk | | |
	A	B	C
Men	3.4	2.7	2.5
Women	5.9	3.4	9.4

A: unadjusted
B: adjusted for age
C: adjusted for age, systolic blood pressure, serum cholesterol, smoking and obesity

analysis age and diabetes appeared to have a significant interaction, the relative risk being appreciably greater in younger than in older age groups.

Hypertension and obesity are known to be more common in diabetics. Hypertriglyceridaemia is the most prominent lipid disorder in diabetics while the prevalence of hypercholesterolaemia is often also increased. Low HDL cholesterol is very common in all type 2 diabetics and in type 1 diabetics with insufficient insulin substitution. In well-controlled type 1 diabetics, HDL cholesterol is often higher than the normal range. The frequency of smoking in diabetics varies and no consistent trend is apparent. All these risk factors are powerful predictors of CHD and hence may explain the excess CHD rates in diabetics. In population studies the relative risk of male and female diabetics dying from CHD has often been shown to decrease after allowing for other risk factors, but in general, the relative risk remains highly significant.[22] In some studies the decrease in relative risk has been greater in women than in men.[18,22] In our prospective study the relative CHD mortality risks hardly changed in men after allowing for other risk factors but increased in women (Table 5.2). The excess CHD mortality in diabetics, therefore, appears to be mediated mainly through factors other than conventional CHD risk factors.

DISCUSSION

The increased CHD morbidity and mortality in diabetics, particularly in women, is well established. Although the detailed information is still somewhat insufficient it may be stated that the excess CHD rates apply to both type 1 and type 2 diseases. The two main unresolved questions are the mechanism by which diabetes increases the risk and why women are especially vulnerable to this risk factor.

Some proportion of the increased CHD risk in diabetics is undoubtedly caused by other risk factors, but a greater proportion of the excess risk seemed to be linked with the disease itself. The degree of hyperglycaemia, altered platelet function and decreased fibrinolytic activity are some factors common in diabetics and they may be potential candidates for explaining the excess risks. Until now the factors were far from clear and much investigation is still necessary.

It has been postulated that female diabetics lack some protective factor which operates in non-diabetic women and allows the well-known sex difference in the morbidity and mortality in CHD. There are, however, hardly any ideas about the nature of this kind of protective factor. Potential protective factors, such as high

HDL cholesterol concentrations and sex-hormone balance, are at the same level in young and middle-aged women with or without diabetes. It may also be postulated, however, that women may be particularly vulnerable to some metabolic risk factors. This kind of sex difference has been shown to operate in hyperuricaemia[23] and hypertriglyceridaemia.[24] Because these metabolic disorders are often also associated with diabetes it is possible that some common risk pathways exist.

From a public health point of view excess CHD morbidity is of limited importance because of the rather low prevalence of the disease. Nevertheless, it is hoped that the problems associated with the observed excess risk for female diabetics will stimulate productive investigations which may further elucidate the pathogenesis and causes for sex difference in CHD.

SUMMARY

Diabetics are specially prone to coronary heart disease (CHD). Obstructive atherosclerotic lesions are undoubtedly more common in diabetics and CHD mortality is much higher than in non-diabetics. Women and men with diabetes are equally affected. Hence the relative resistance of female diabetics to CHD is lost when compared with women without diabetes. Conventional CHD risk factors explain only a small fraction of the excess CHD rates in diabetics. The effect of diabetes seemed to be mainly mediated by factors connected with the metabolic disorder itself.

REFERENCES

1 Pyörälä K, Laakso M. Macrovascular disease in diabetes mellitus. In: Mann JI, Pyörälä K, Teuscher A, eds. Diabetes in epidemiological perspective. Edinburgh, London, Melbourne, New York: Churchill Livingstone, 1983: 183–247.
2 West KM. Epidemiology of diabetes and its vascular lesions. New York: Elsevier, 1978.
3 National Diabetes Data Group. Classification and diagnosis of diabetes mellitus and other categories of glucose intolerance. Diabetes 1979; 28: 1039–57.
4 WHO Expert Committee on diabetes mellitus. Second Report. Technical Report Series 646 Geneva, World Health Organization, 1980.
5 Reunanen A. Akerblom HK, Käär ML. Prevalence and ten year (1970–79) incidence of insulin-dependent diabetes mellitus in children and adolescents in Finland. Acta Paediatr Scand 1982; 71: 893–9.
6 Garcia MJ, McNamara PM, Gordon T, Kannel WB. Morbidity and mortality in diabetics in the Framingham population. Sixteen year follow-up study. Diabetes 1974; 23: 105–11.
7 Barrett-Connor E. The prevalence of diabetes mellitus in an adult community as determined by history of fasting hyperglycemia. Am J Epidemiol 1980; 111: 705–12.
8 Reunanen A. Prevalence and incidence of type 2 diabetes in Finland. Acta Endocrinol (Copenh) 1984; suppl 262: 31–5.
9 Bradley RF. Cardiovascular disease. In: Marble A, White P, Bradley RF, Krall LP, eds. Joslin's diabetes mellitus. 11th ed. Philadelphia: Lea and Febiger, 1971: 417–77.
10 Robertson WB, Strong JP. Atherosclerosis in persons with hypertension and diabetes mellitus. Lab Invest 1968; 18: 538–51.
11 Zdanov VS, Vihert AM. Atherosclerosis and diabetes mellitus. Bull WHO 1976; 53: 547–53.
12 Keen H, Jarrett RJ. The WHO multinational study of vascular disease in diabetes: 2. Macrovascular disease prevalence. Diabetes Care 1979; 2: 187–95.
13 Uusitupa M. Coronary heart disease and left ventricular performance in newly diagnosed non-insulin-dependent diabetics. Kuopio: University of Kuopio, 1983. (Thesis)

[14] Marks HH, Krall LP. Onset, course, prognosis, and mortality in diabetes mellitus. In: Marble A, White P, Bradley RF, Krall LP, eds. Joslin's diabetes mellitus. 11th ed. Philadelphia: Lea and Febiger, 1971: 209–54.

[15] Kannel WB, McGee DL. Diabetes and glucose tolerance as risk factors for cardiovascular disease: the Framingham study. Diabetes Care 1979; 2: 120–6.

[16] Heyden S, Heiss G, Bartel AG, Hames CG. Sex differences in coronary mortality among diabetics in Evans County, Georgia. J Chronic Dis 1980; 33: 265–73.

[17] Jarrett RJ, McCartney P, Keen H. The Bedford Survey: ten year mortality rates in newly diagnosed diabetics, borderline diabetics and normoglycaemic controls and risk indices for coronary heart disease in borderline diabetics. Diabetologia 1982; 22: 79–84.

[18] Barrett-Connor E, Wingard DL. Sex differential in ischemic heart disease mortality in diabetics: a prospective population-based study. Am J Epidemiol 1983; 118: 489–96.

[19] Soler NG, Bennett MA, Pentecost BL, Fitzgerald MG, Malins JM. Myocardial infarction in diabetics. Q J Med 1975; 44: 125–32.

[20] Królewski AS, Czyżyk A, Janeczko D, Kopczyński J. Mortality from cardiovascular diseases among diabetics. Diabetologia 1977; 13: 345–50.

[21] Panzram G, Zabel-Langhennig R. Prognosis of diabetes mellitus in a geographically defined population. Diabetologia 1981; 20: 587–91.

[22] Kannel WB, McGee DL. Diabetes and cardiovascular disease. The Framingham Study. JAMA 1979; 241: 2035–8.

[23] Reunanen A, Takkunen H, Knekt P, Aromaa A. Hyperuricemia as a risk factor for cardiovascular mortality. Acta Med Scand 1982; suppl 668: 49–59.

[24] Gordon T, Castelli WP, Hjortland MC, Kannel WB, Dawber TR. Diabetes, blood lipids, and the role of obesity in coronary heart disease risk for women. The Framingham Study. Ann Intern Med 1977; 87: 393–7.

Discussion on Chapter 5

Oliver
In the Edinburgh-Stockholm study in men aged 40 the most important difference between the coronary-prone Scottish population and the less coronary-prone Swedish population was that the insulin response to a standard glucose load was quite different, with the Scots having a greater insulin response to glucose. This also occurred earlier and the area under the curve was greater. What is the relationship between insulin response to a glucose load and coronary predisposition?

Nikkilä
Nobody knows why these people have hyperinsulinaemia. There are no good studies—for example, it is not explained by obesity.

Wynn
Apart from the hyperinsulinaemia another observation in the Edinburgh-Stockholm study was the prevalence of high triglycerides. I was surprised when Dr Nikkilä said that raised triglycerides are not risk factors. In our experience we find raised triglycerides to be an independent risk factor. We also have confirmed that hyperinsulinaemia is a risk factor in a group of male atherosclerotics. They were selected beforehand as having apparently normal glucose metabolism and normal cholesterol levels. Nevertheless, that group of individuals show hyperinsulinaemia when tested against controls.

In the presentation there was a surprising finding that most of the excess mortality in the diabetic women was in the insulin-requiring diabetics. This is contrary to the experience of a lot of people.

Reunanen
Yes, if we are looking at risk ratios in women with maturity-onset diabetes treated by diet alone it is nearly 1 but among women treated with tablets it is about 2.

Shapiro
It could be an artefact because insulin-requiring diabetics are really diabetic; people who simply have been diagnosed may or may not be diabetic; people who are getting tablets probably are diabetic.

Wynn
I suppose the explanation of this surprising finding is that the insulin-requiring diabetics have a more severe form of the disease and have had it longer, probably from under the age of 30 and they probably die between 50 and 60. There is no agreed definition of maturity-onset diabetes.

What risk is posed by impaired glucose tolerance short of clinical diabetes? If you did full glucose tolerance tests with insulin measurements in your control subjects you would find a high prevalence of undiagnosed diabetes and among them a higher-than-normal incidence of coronary heart disease. Those undiagnosed cases are altering the risk ratio so you have not got a true non-diabetic control population, just a population in which there are a number of undiagnosed diabetics.

You are then comparing the groups with a group of individuals in whom diabetes has been diagnosed. Often we found that when a patient comes into hospital with a coronary that is when the diagnosis of diabetes is made. That individual has probably had diabetes for 10 or 20 years in an undiagnosed form.

Reunanen
In our study the diagnostic criteria depended on glucose tolerance tests but without insulin measurements. Over 50 000 tests were made.

6. Oral contraception: hormonal influences on blood pressure

R.J. Weir and J.I.S. Robertson

HIGH DOSE OESTROGEN-PROGESTAGEN COMBINATIONS

Studies of blood pressure changes associated with oral contraception were initially based on the 50–100 μg oestrogen combinations. In a large UK Multicentre study by the Royal College of General Practitioners,[1] 23 000 pill-users were compared with a control group of non-users. The incidence of hypertension diagnosed after 5 years was 2.6 times higher in the users than in the non-users and appeared to increase with the duration of oral contraceptive use and the age of the taker. Similar data were obtained in the United States[2] when 13 358 women were studied for 3 years, with an incidence of hypertension in the users five times greater than non-users. Workers studying other populations and using varying criteria for the diagnosis of hypertension, reported an incidence of hypertension of between 1% and 15% among oral contraceptive users.[3-5] Rare cases of malignant-phase hypertension have been described.[6]

A general effect on blood pressure in women taking 50–100 μg oestrogen combinations has also been found. In a prospective controlled study of 186 women over 2 years, systemic pressure rose in 164 women (mean rise 7.7 mm Hg) and diastolic in 150 women (mean rise 4.2 mm Hg) with no significant change in women using intra-uterine devices or barrier methods of contraception.[7]

LOW DOSE OESTROGEN-PROGESTAGEN COMBINATIONS

The effect of lower dose oestrogen-progestagen oral contraceptives on blood pressure has been more controversial. A cross-sectional population study in London showed the blood pressure to be higher in women taking 30 μg oestrogen-containing pills than in those taking 50 μg oestrogen combinations.[8] However, in a prospective study of 58 normotensive women, combined oral contraceptives containing 30 μg ethinyloestradiol plus 150 μg levonorgestrel showed no significant effect on blood pressure after 3 years, compared with a significant rise in blood pressure in women taking 50 μg oestrogen combination for the same time.[9]

We have recently completed a prospective, controlled study of blood pressure changes in women taking oral contraceptives containing 30 μg ethinyloestradiol plus 150 μg levonorgestrel and 30 μg ethinyloestradiol plus 2 mg ethynodiol diacetate.[10] Each woman had a routine medical and gynaecological examination before entry. Any with a blood pressure of 140/90 mm Hg or more were excluded. Blood pressure was measured by a research nurse, using an Elag-Köln automatic blood pressure recorder with printout, to reduce observer error. Blood pressure was taken after the women had sat quietly for at least 2 minutes, with the arm resting horizontally. The lowest of three readings was used for statistical analysis. Further measurements were made under the same standardised conditions at intervals of 2, 4, 6, 9, 12, 18 and 24 months.

Table 6.1 Mean systolic and diastolic blood pressure ($\pm$sem) at entry and after 1 year.

Group	n	Entry SBP	DBP	1 year SBP	DBP
IUD/Controls	143	112.5±3.0	73.5±2.5	109.5±3.1	*68.2±2.4
Ethinyl oestradiol 30 μg + Levonorgestrel 150 μg	137	106.6±2.2	68.0±2.0	*113.0±2.3	*70.7±2.5
Ethinyl oestradiol 30 μg + Ethynodiol diacetate 2 mg	91	112.0±2.0	67.5±2.3	**118.2±2.6	*70.5±2.4
Norethisterone 350 μg	43	110.0±3.5	75.9±4.0	*104.7±3.6	*71.5±3.0
Norgestrel 75 μg	30	111.6±3.5	75.0±3.5	106.0±3.0	*67.9±3.0
Ethynodiol diacetate 500 μg	21	108.7±4.0	74.5±4.5	112.4±4.5	73.5±3.5
Norethisterone oenanthate 200 mg im	20	108.7±3.3	69.9±4.0	105.4±3.9	66.5±4.9

*p<0.05, *p<0.01, **p<0.001

Table 6.1 shows the changes in mean systolic and diastolic blood pressure in the 485 women followed up for 1 year. It will be seen that a significant increase in both systolic and diastolic blood pressure occurred in the groups taking oral contraceptives containing ethinyloestradiol combined with levonorgestrel or ethynodiol diacetate. In contrast, the control group and progestagen-only groups showed no change or a fall in blood pressure.

After 2 years, mean systolic pressure had risen by 7.0 mm Hg and 7.2 mm Hg in the two oestrogen groups (Fig. 6.1). Diastolic pressure rose by 4.2 mm Hg and 4.1 mm Hg during the same period (p < 0.05). No significant change occurred in the groups using intra-uterine devices, barrier methods or progestagen alone.

The incidence of hypertension in women taking low dose oestrogen-progestagen oral contraceptives is not known. Malignant-phase hypertension may occur,[11] as described in the following cases.

Case 1

This patient was nulliparous with no family history of hypertension. She was overweight but a non-smoker. Her first recorded blood pressure was 150/80 mm Hg obtained when she sought contraceptive advice from her local family planning clinic. She was prescribed levonogestrel 0.15 mg and ethinyloestradiol 0.03 mg (Microgynon 30).

8 weeks later she was admitted to a Canadian hospital with a 2 week history of malaise, nausea and visual deterioration. Blood pressure on admission was 244/170 mm Hg and fundoscopy revealed bilateral haemorrhages, exudates and papilloede-

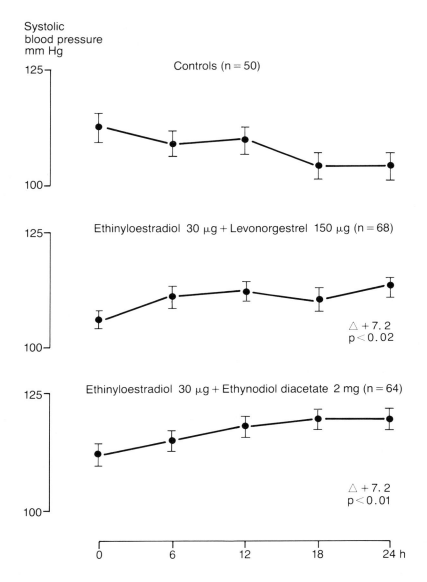

Fig. 6.1 Mean systolic blood pressure (±SEM) after 2 years in women taking oestrogen-progestagen oral contraceptives and in controls.

ma. Plasma sodium was 139 mmol/l, potassium 3.4 mmol/l, chloride 97 mmol/l and urea 14 mmol/l. Before treatment could be instituted she developed a grand mal seizure which subsided rapidly and spontaneously. A sodium nitroprusside infusion was started which reduced her pressure to 140/90 mm Hg over the next 24 hours. Further investigation was not performed and she was transferred to this department 1 week later for additional assessment. Blood pressure was 140/90 mm Hg on propranolol 240 mg daily and methyldopa 750 mg daily. Urine contained no blood, glucose, protein or organisms. Creatinine clearance was 62 ml/min. Neither chest X-ray nor ECG showed evidence of cardiac enlargement.

Intravenous pyelography revealed normal kidney outlines, but the right kidney was distinctly smaller than the left (12.4 cm as compared with 15 cm in the long axis). Pyelographic density was increased on the right suggesting right renal artery stenosis. Renal arteriography, however, showed no evidence of main or branch renal artery stenosis. In view of the abnormalities noted on intravenous pyelogram (IVP), and despite the normal arteriogram, further assessment of renal function was undertaken. Bilateral ureteric catheter studies showed reduced urine flow and clearances of para-aminohippurate (PAH) and creatinine from the right kidney. Urinary concentrations of creatinine and PAH were higher on the right. Isotope renogram confirmed reduced blood flow via the right kidney. Bilateral renal vein sampling with simultaneous arterial sampling showed consistently higher active renin concentration in the right renal vein (mean of three samples 102 μU/ml) than in aortic (mean 69 μU/ml) or left renal venous plasma (mean 85 μU/ml). It was considered that these findings could have been due to predominantly right-sided intrarenal arteriolar damage, either the consequence of the malignant phase or contraceptive-induced arteriolitis. She was discharged on atenolol 100 mg daily, methyldopa 1500 mg daily and bendrofluazide 5 mg daily, and subsequently changed to atenolol 200 mg daily, bendrofluazide 10 mg daily and prazosin 8 mg daily.

Although the retinal lesions have resolved, control in the subsequent 3 years has been variable, with blood pressures ranging from 138/94 to 200/120 mm Hg. Compliance with treatment is almost certainly erratic.

Case 2

This unmarried woman had consistently normal blood pressure recordings of up to 120/70 mm Hg during her only pregnancy when she was 17 years old. She went to full term and delivery was normal. Her last blood pressure reading, immediately post-partum, was 150/90 mm Hg. One month later she was prescribed levonorgestrel 0.25 mg and ethinyloestradiol 0.03 mg (Eugynon 30) which was continued over the next 2 years without further blood pressure recordings being made. She was a non-smoker and was not overweight.

She then complained of malaise, headaches, nausea, weight loss and blurred vision. 2 months after the onset of these symptoms she was admitted to another hospital with a blood pressure of 260/160 mm Hg. Fundoscopy revealed bilateral haemorrhages, exudates and papilloedema. Plasma sodium was 113 mmol/l, potassium 3.3 mmol/l, chloride 89 mmol/l and urea 6.6 mmol/l. Diazoxide 300 mg by intravenous bolus, frusemide 40 mg orally and methyldopa 500 mg orally were prescribed, but reduced blood pressure to only 200/120 mm Hg 6 hours later. Diazoxide 300 mg and methyldopa 500 mg were administered, both intravenously. 10 hours later she was in a coma with blood pressure 140/90 mm Hg. She was then transferred to specialist neurological care where the diagnosis of brain damage consequent to diminished cerebral perfusion was made.

She was later admitted to this department with blood pressures in the range 120/70–160/90 mm Hg on atenolol 100 mg daily, frusemide 40 mg daily and hydralazine 150 mg daily. She remained disorientated and irrational. Serum urea and electrolytes were normal with creatinine clearance 44 ml/min. Chest X-ray showed cardiac enlargement and the ECG evidence of left ventricular hypertrophy. IVP was normal. Her mental impairment was such that further investigation was not considered appropriate. The retinal lesions resolved slowly.

There seems little doubt, therefore, that oral contraceptives containing 30 μg oestrogen plus progestagen cause a rise in blood pressure in most women, and in rare cases may induce malignant phase hypertension.

TRIPHASIC OESTROGEN-PROGESTAGEN ORAL CONTRACEPTIVES

It has been suggested that the new triphasic oral contraceptives will be less likely to affect blood pressure because of the lower overall monthly intake of progestagen. In two studies[12,13] no significant change in blood pressure was found in women using triphasic preparations. In another study,[14] however, two patients were reported to have developed hypertension while taking a triphasic pill containing a mean daily dose of 32.4 μg ethinyloestradiol and 91.7 μg levonorgestrel.

PROGESTAGEN ALONE

Table 6.1 shows the changes in blood pressure over 1 year in women taking norethisterone 350 μg, norgestrel 75 μg, ethynodiol diacetate 500 μg and norethisterone oenanthate 200 μg im. No significant increase in blood pressure occurred in any of these groups, and this was confirmed after a 2 year follow-up.[10] These results are in keeping with previous studies.[15-17]

To date, there is no evidence that progestagen given alone to normotensive women will cause hypertension, but it has been shown that progestagens may cause a small rise in blood pressure in women with previous hypertension induced by an oestrogen-progestagen combination.[18]

THE ROLE OF THE OESTROGEN AND PROGESTAGEN COMPONENTS IN THE RISE OF BLOOD PRESSURE

In the large study conducted by the Royal College of General Practitioners[1] the incidence of hypertension appeared to be related to the dose of progestagen but not to the dose of oestrogen. Nevertheless, this was a non-standardised study in which the participating doctors were asked to report the diagnosis of hypertension based on their own individual criteria and the data must therefore be interpreted with some reservations. In the standardised, controlled, prospective Glasgow study,[7] no relationship was found between the rise in blood pressure and the type or dose of progestagen used. In a more recent study comparing different doses of norethisterone acetate (1.0, 2.5, 3.0 and 4.0 mg) combined with 50 μg ethinyloestradiol, no relationship was found with the incidence of hypertension.[19] As already stated, there is no evidence to date that progestagens given alone will affect blood pressure in previously normotensive women.[10,15-17]

An increase in systolic blood pressure has been shown during intravenous infusion of oestrogens,[20] and administration of oral oestrogens—especially ethinyl-oestradiol in doses equivalent to those in the combined contraceptive pill—caused significant increases in blood pressure.[16] The use of smaller doses of oestrogen did not, however, cause a significant change in blood pressure.[21] It seems likely, therefore, that it is the oestrogen component which is the main culprit, but perhaps there is a synergistic action with the associated progestagen.

POSSIBLE MECHANISMS FOR THE RISE IN BLOOD PRESSURE

The mechanism leading to the rise in arterial pressure induced by oestrogen-progestagen contraceptives has not been identified. Possible factors include increased mineralocorticoid activity and changes in the renin-angiotensin system.

The pressor effect of angiotensin II is enhanced by sodium retention and diminished by sodium depletion.[22] It is therefore important, in assessing the effect of any changes in plasma angotensin II, to relate these (if possible) to concurrent body sodium content. We have examined the renin-angiotensin-aldosterone system together with whole body sodium and potassium composition in women with hypertension while taking oral contraceptives, and compared these measurements with those made in age-matched women with essential hypertension. The methods have been described in detail elsewhere.[23]

One group of patients consisted of six women who presented with hypertension while taking a combined oestrogen-progestagen oral contraceptive (30–50 μg oestrogen). The second group consisted of age-matched women with essential hypertension.

After withdrawing the oral contraceptive, arterial pressure fell spontaneously in five of the six patients within 24 months. In the sixth patient (patient 5), blood pressure also returned to normal but oxprenolol had been prescribed after the conclusion of investigations because of concurrent angina. There were no significant differences between the two groups in age, mean body weight or systolic and diastolic pressure.

Plasma renin-substrate was significantly higher ($p < 0.01$) in the women taking oral contraceptives (1.39 ± 0.23 μmol/l) than in essential hypertensives (0.55 ± 0.04 μmol/l) (Table 6.2). The mean value for the oral contraceptive users was above the upper limit of the normal range. The plasma active renin concentration, by contrast, was closely similar in the two groups (respectively 27.0 ± 5.0 μU/ml and 27.0 ± 8.7 μU/ml). Both values lie in the middle of the normal range. In accordance with the plasma renin and substrate measurements, plasma angiotensin II was significantly raised ($p < 0.02$) in the women taking oral contraceptives (38.0 ± 5 pmol/l) in comparison with the women with essential hypertension (20.0 ± 4 pmol/l). the former mean value lies above the upper limit of normal for our laboratory. It is interesting that overall there was a significant correlation between the product of active renin and renin-substrate concentration and angiotensin II ($r = 0.68$, $p<0.05$).

The plasma aldosterone concentration did not differ significantly between the contraceptive users (378 ± 36 pmol/l) and the patients with essential hypertension

(373±72 pmol/l). In the oral contraceptive users and in the essential hypertensive patients respectively, mean total body sodium was 100.1±4.7 (SEM) % and 94.5±1.4%; total body potassium 97.7±6.0% and 104.6±1.4%. There was no significant difference in these measurements between the two groups. Similarly, mean plasma sodium and potassium did not differ significantly between the two groups (respectively 138.0±0.9 SEM mmol/l and 140.0±0.5 mmol/l; 4.3±0.1 mmol/l and 4.1±0.1 mmol/l).

Table 6.2 Measurements of the renin-angiotensin system and total body sodium and potassium in oral contraceptive users and essential hypertensives.

Patient number	Renin-substrate (μmol/l)	Renin (μU/ml)	AngiotensinII (pmol/l)	Aldosterone (pmol/l)	Total body sodium (%)	Total body potassium (%)
Oral contraceptive users						
1	0.87	37	40	440	113.1	–
2	1.11	38	28	410	93	89.6
3	1.12	15	38	500	103.3	103.2
4	1.96	13	51	280	102.8	116.8
5	2.22	45	50	360	107.7	97.4
6	1.05	14	23	280	80.7	81.3
Mean	1.38	27.0	38.0	378.3	100.1	97.7
Essential hypertensives						
7	0.51	15	22	140	93.6	107.8
8	0.65	31	16	610	96.1	99.5
9	–	66	37	550	94.4	101.6
10	0.44	5	12	330	89.8	107.9
11	0.52	16	12	330	99.9	104.6
12	0.61	29	23	280	93.2	106.2
Mean	0.55	27.0	20.0	373.3	94.5	104.6

Plasma renin-substrate concentration has consistently been found to be increased during oral contraceptive usage,[24-28] and this finding is confirmed in the present study. Plasma renin activity, a measurement dependent simultaneously on renin and substrate concentrations, has been variously found to be increased or unchanged.[24,29-31]

In oral contraceptive users, Skinner et al[24] described a concurrent increase in renin-substrate and depression of renin concentration together with plasma renin activity twice that found in normal subjects. They hypothesised that the rise in renin-substrate brought the renin-substrate reaction closer to its maximum velocity, thus increasing angiotensin II production which then had a direct suppressive effect on the renal release of renin. Doubt remains whether the accelerated rate of the renin-renin-substrate reaction depends only on renin-substrate concentration[24,28] or upon an increase in maximal velocity of the reaction[32] in addition to the renin-substrate concentration. However, multiple forms of renin-substrate have been described when production is stimulated by oestrogen or corticosteroids[33] so these different forms of plasma renin-substrate may variously influence the rate of renin reaction in several hypertensive states.

In the present study, despite the consistently higher renin-substrate values in the hypertensive women taking oral contraceptives, the plasma concentration of active renin was not suppressed, being similar to values found in essential hypertension. Both values were in the middle of the normal range. Not surprisingly, therefore, plasma angiotensin II was significantly higher in the women taking the pill, and the mean value for the group was slightly above the upper limit of normal. Cain et al[25] also found a significant rise in whole blood angiotension II with oral contraceptive use, while Weir et al[26] reported a slight but insignificant rise in mean plasma angiotensin II concentration.

In the contraceptive users, mean total body sodium was slightly but insignificantly higher than in the essential hypertensive group, with values near normal; conversely, total body potassium was slightly but insignificantly lower. Mean values of body sodium and potassium content do not differ from normal in essential hypertension.[34] Exchangeable and total body sodium, however, are positively correlated with arterial pressure[34,35] in essential hypertension. Body sodium content tends to be low in younger essential hypertensives, and to increase in older patients with more severe hypertension.[35]

The slightly (albeit insignificantly) lower total body sodium content in the present group of young women with essential hypertension is therefore consistent with the findings in the larger series. In the same context, there are known to be age-related falls in plasma renin, angiotensin II and aldosterone in normal subjects and in patients with essential hypertension.[36,37] The age ranges of our present patients with essential hypertension and those using oral contraceptives were wide but similar in the two groups.

The present findings are therefore consistent with the concept that the raised blood pressure in the women taking the oestrogen-progestagen pill may be at least partly due to an increase in plasma angiotensin II in relation to total body sodium. The normality of body sodium and potassium content provides no evidence in support of the view that the raised blood pressure depends on increased mineralocorticoid activity.[38] Our findings, however, are in agreement with those of Cain et al[25] who found that the contraceptive pill raised circulating angiotensin II. They are also in accord with the indirect evidence of Streeten et al[39] who demonstrated, by infusing saralasin, an acute reduction in blood pressure in women hypertensives while taking oral contraceptives, although this was not confirmed in another study.[40]

REFERENCES

[1]Royal College of General Practitioners' Oral Contraception Study. Effect on hypertension and benign breast disease of progestagen component in combined oral contraceptives. Lancet 1977; 1: 624.

[2]Fisch IR, Frank J. Oral contraceptives and blood pressure. JAMA 1977; 237: 2499-503.

[3]Wallace MR. Oral contraceptives and severe hypertension. Aust NZ J Med 1971; 1: 49-52.

[4]Clezy TM, Foy BN, Hodge RL, Lumbers ER. Oral contraceptives and hypertension. An epidemiological survey. Br Heart J 1972; 34: 1238-43.

[5]Stern MP, Brown BW, Haskell WL, Farquhar JW, Wehrle CL, Wood PDS. Cardiovascular risk and use of estrogens or estrogen-progestagen combinations. Stanford Three-Community Study. J Am Med Assoc 1976; 235: 811-5.

[6]Dunn FG, Jones JV, Fife R. Malignant hypertension associated with use of oral contraceptives. Br Heart J 1975; 37: 336-8.

[7]Weir RJ, Briggs E, Mack A, Naismith L, Taylor L, Wilson E. Blood pressure in women taking oral contraceptives. Br Med J 1974; 1: 533-5.

[8]Meade TW, Haines AP, North WRS, Chakrabarti R, Howarth DJ, Stirling Y. Haemostatic, lipid, and blood-pressure profiles of women on oral contraceptives containing 50 μg or 30 μg oestrogen. Lancet 1977; 2: 948-51.

[9]Briggs M, Briggs M. Oestrogen content of oral contraceptives. Lancet 1977; 2: 1233.

[10]Weir RJ, Wilson ESB, Cruikshank J, McMaster M. Effects on blood pressure of low dose oestrogen and progestagen only oral contraceptives. J Hypertension 1983; 1(suppl 2): 100–1.

[11]Hodsman GP, Robertson JIS, Semple PF, Mackay A. Malignant hypertension and oral contraceptives: four cases with two due to the 30 μg oestrogen pill. Eur Heart J 1982; 3: 255–9.

[12]Gaspard UK, Deville JL, Dubois MH. Clinical experience with triphasic oral contraceptives (Trigynon) in six hundred cycles. In: Haspels AA, Rolland R, eds. Benefits and risks of hormonal contraception, England: MJP Press, 1982: 61–77.

[13]Zador G. Clinical performance of a triphasic administration of ethinyl oestradiol and levonorgestrel in comparison with the 30+150 μg fixed-dose regime. In: Haspels AA, Rolland R, eds. Benefits and risks of hormonal contraception. England: MJP Press, 1982: 43–55.

[14]Carlborg L. Acceptability of low dose oral contraceptives: results of a randomised Swedish multicenter study comparing a triphasic (Trionetta) and a fixed dose combination (Neovletta). In: Haspels AA, Rolland R, eds. Benefits and risks of hormonal contraception. England: MJP Press, 1982: 78–90.

[15]Mackay EV, Khoo SK, Adam RR. Contraception with a six-monthly injection of progestogen. Part 1. Effects on blood pressure, body weight and uterine bleeding pattern, side-effects, efficacy and acceptability. Aust NZ J Obstet Gynaecol 1971; 11: 148–55.

[16]Spellacy WN, Birk SA. The effect of intra-uterine devices, oral contraceptives, estrogens, and progestogens on blood pressure. Am J Obstet Gynecol 1972; 112: 912–9.

[17]Hawkins DF, Benster B. A comparative study of three low dose progestogens, chlormadinone acetate, megestrol acetate and norethisterone, as oral contraceptives. Br J Obstet Gynaecol 1977; 84: 708–13.

[18]Weir RJ. Effect on blood pressure of changing from high to low dose steroid preparations in women with oral contraceptive induced hypertension. Scott Med J 1982; 27: 212–5.

[19]Meade TW, Greenberg G, Thompson SG. Progestogens and cardiovascular reactions associated with oral contraceptives and a comparison of the safety of 50- and 30-μg oestrogen preparations. Br Med J 1980; 280: 1157–61.

[20]Lim YL, Lumbers ER, Walters WAW, Whelan RF. Effects of oestrogens on the human circulatin. Br J Obstet Gynaecol 1970; 77: 349–55.

[21]Gow S, MacGillivray I. Metabolic, hormonal and vascular changes after synthetic oestrogen therapy in oophorectomized women. Br Med J 1971; 2: 73–7.

[22]Oelkers W, Brown JJ, Fraser R, Lever AF, Morton JJ, Robertson JIS. Sensitization of the adrenal cortex to angiotensin II in sodium-deplete man. Circ Res 1974; 34: 69–77.

[23]McAreavey D, Cumming AMM, Boddy K et al. The renin-angiotensin system and total body sodium and potassium in hypertensive women taking oestrogen-progestagen oral contraceptives. Clin Endocrinol (Oxf) 1983; 18: 111–8.

[24]Skinner SL, Lumbers ER, Symonds EM. Alteration by oral contraceptives of normal menstrual changes in plasma renin activity, concentration and substrate. Clin Sci 1969; 36: 67–76.

[25]Cain MD, Walters WA, Catt KJ. Effects of oral contraceptive therapy on the renin-angiotensin system. J Clin Endocrinol Metab 1971; 33: 671–6.

[26]Weir RJ, Tree M, McElwee G. Changes in blood pressure and in plasma renin, renin-substrate and angiotensin II concentrations in women taking contraceptive steroids. In: Snow RO, ed. Proceedings of the Fourth International Congress of Endocrinology. Amsterdam: Excerpta Medica, 1972: 1019–25.

[27]Tree M. Measurement of plasma renin-substrate in man. J Endocrinol 1973; 56: 159a–71a.

[28]Gould AB, DeWolf R, Goodman S, Onesti G, Swartz C. Kinetic studies of the human renin and human substrate reaction. Biochem Med 1980; 24: 321–6.

[29]Weinberger MH, Collins RD, Dowdy AJ, Nokes GW, Luetscher JA. Hypertension induced by oral contraceptives containing estrogen and gestagen. Effects on plasma renin activity and aldosterone excretion. Ann Intern Med 1969; 71: 891–902.

[30]Saruta T, Saade GA, Kaplan NM. A possible mechanism for hypertension induced by oral contraceptives. Diminished feedback suppression of renin release. Arch Intern Med 1970; 126: 621–6.

[31]Crane MG, Harris JJ, Winsor W. Hypertension, oral contraceptive agents, and conjugated estrogens. Ann Intern Med 1971; 74: 13–21.

[32]McDonald WJ, Cohen EL, Lucas CP, Conn JW. Renin-renin substrate kinetic constants in the plasma of normal and estrogen-treated humans. J Clin Endocrinol Metab 1977; 45: 1297–304.

[33]Eggena P, Hidaka H, Barrett JD, Sambhi MP. Multiple forms of human plasma renin substrate. J Clin Invest 1978; 62: 367–72.

[34]Beretta-Piccoli C, Davies DL, Boddy K et al. Relation of arterial pressure with exchangeable and total body potassium in essential hypertension. Clin Sci 1981; 61(suppl 7): 81–4.

62

[35]Lever AF, Beretta-Piccoli C, Brown JJ, Davies DL, Fraser R, Robertson JIS. Sodium and potassium in essential hypertension. Br Med J 1981; 283: 463–8.

[36]Padfield PL, Beevers DG, Brown JJ et al. Is low-renin hypertension a stage in the development of essential hypertension or a diagnostic entity? Lancet 1975; 1: 548–50.

[37]Zadik ZVI, Kowarski AA. Normal integrated concentration of aldosterone and plasma renin activity: effect of age. J Clin Endocrinol Metab 1980; 50: 867–9.

[38]Laragh JH. Oral contraceptive-induced hypertension—Nine years later. Am J Obstet Gynecol 1976; 126: 141–7.

[39]Streeten DHP, Anderson GH, Dalakos TG. Angiotensin blockade: Its clinical significance. Am J Med 1976; 60: 817–24.

[40]Broughton-Pipkin F, Hunter JC, Oats J, Symonds M. Hypertension and oral contraceptives. Br Med J 1978; 2: 278.

Discussion on Chapter 6

Oliver

The Royal College of General Practitioners reported a mild hypertensive effect with progesterone-only pills. What do you advise for a woman who is mildly hypertensive and who requires an oral contraceptive? Should she have a progestagen-only pill?

Weir

The problem during the Royal College of General Practitioners' study was that the blood pressure measurements in that study were taken by a large number of doctors in a large number of different settings using different criteria for hypertension. They found that women taking the pills with a higher dosage of progestagen did appear to have a higher incidence of hypertension, but I think that there are some qualifications about the study. In response to your question, if a woman has high blood pressure I personally would prefer not to put her on a contraceptive pill at all. If there are strong reasons for giving her a contraceptive pill, I would have no hesitation, with present knowledge, in giving her a progestagen preparation.

Beaumont J.-L.

Is there any relation between this mild elevation in blood pressure in women taking the pill and an increased risk of cardiovascular disease? Alternatively, do the grave cases of hypertensive disease induced by pills explain the increased risk of cardiovascular disease among women taking the pill?

Weir

These women developed a rise in blood pressure over a period of 3 years. Some women may take the pill for 5, 10 or 15 years, or more. Over that period many of these women may show an increase in both systolic and diastolic blood pressure, into a range which, according to the Framingham data and according to the Society of Actuaries' data, would put them at risk of cardiovascular disease. We have to take into account the fact that, in addition to the blood pressure changes, these women have changes in glucose equal metabolism, insulin secretion, changes in coagulation and perhaps other risk factors. Blood pressure, however, is one factor possibly more important in relation to cerebrovascular disease than to myocardial infarction.

Shapiro

What about the cases appearing in the first year of use?

Weir

One would expect the women showing marked rises in blood pressure to be at risk not only from cerebral vascular disease but from cardiac failure, angina pectoris and myocardial infarction.

Shapiro

We know when oral contraceptive use is stopped there is a very sudden drop in the risk for both cerebral vascular disease and for myocardial infarction—and indeed for thrombosis—throughout the body. This suggests that one strong effect of oral contraceptives is on clotting mechanisms. In addition, there is the concern that oral contraceptives have a long-term effect on blood pressure, and blood glucose levels and lipid patterns, which are also adverse. On the whole I think the epidemiological data suggest that for the risk of both stroke and myocardial infarction the effect of hypertension induced by oral contraceptives is modest.

Weir

I agree that these other factors are important. It is also important to realise that the blood pressure will usually fall fairly quickly after the woman stops the pill, within a few weeks or months, but sometimes it may take longer.

Vedin

The response to hormonal manipulation in the patients who have actually developed coronary or other arteriosclerotic disease may be different. We might be dealing with a subpopulation having a different response. This view applies also to Dr Nikkilä's talk.

Bengtsson

Do you consider that there is a normal distribution of blood pressure change while taking contraceptive pills or do few women increase their blood pressure very much?

Weir

The blood pressure changes show a smooth curve which is shifted to the right. There is no specific subgroup of women in which a large rise in blood pressure occurs while the majority remains normal.

Robertson

We wanted to make the point that there were some women who had an acute and very severe rise in blood pressure and who were therefore very sensitive to the pressor effects of oral contraceptives. I think it is not surprising that some of these who showed a very acute rise in pressure suffered severe complications such as the malignant phase. Fortunately, such cases are rare. Most women going on to the pill sustain only a very mild elevation of blood pressure and of course this carries much less risk of cardiovascular complications, at least in the short term.

7. Type A behaviour, employment status, and coronary heart disease in women—a review

S.G. Haynes

INTRODUCTION

During the past 30 years the number of women in the labour force has risen sharply. The growing participation of women in the work place and in higher status jobs has brought fears that women will lose their survival advantage over men, and will have increasingly higher mortality from coronary heart disease (CHD) over time. One basis for these fears is the undocumented assumption that employment in higher status jobs elicits type A behaviour which, in turn, enhances the development or progression of CHD.

The purpose of the present paper is to review and evaluate the accumulated data related to type A behaviour, employment status, and CHD in women. In 1978, a distinguished National Heart, Lung and Blood Institute (NHLBI) panel of biomedical and behavioural scientists concluded that the association between the type A behaviour pattern and coronary incidence had been shown only for a demographically restricted subpopulation—namely, middle-class and upper-class men over the age of 39 years.[1] Studies were proposed for particularly deserving groups such as people working in less prestigious occupations and for women employed outside the home.[1] Particular focus will be given in this paper to the growing number of papers on type A behaviour in women published since the 1978 conference.

The first section of the paper assesses the features of type A behaviour that apply to women, and presents the distribution of the behaviour pattern by age and employment groups. A review of the coronary endpoint data from prospective and case-control studies as well as cross-sectional angiographic studies follows. The third section evaluates the evidence relating type A behaviour to the standard coronary risk factors. The fourth section summarises the recently explored topics of employment status, family responsibilities, and CHD rates in women. The final section highlights several directions for future research.

ASSESSMENT AND DISTRIBUTION OF TYPE A BEHAVIOUR IN WOMEN

The type A behaviour pattern was first described by Friedman and Rosenman among men aged 39 and over.[2] Type A men were described as intensively aggressive, competitive, ambitious, and driven by a chronic sense of time urgency. Hostility was also a component of type A behaviour.[3] The extreme type A man was chronically involved in an almost endless struggle to achieve poorly defined goals against all odds and in less and less time. The type A individual is work-oriented, preoccupied with deadlines, and the behaviour is enhanced by competitive work environments.

There are four common methods for assessing type A behaviour: the structured interview (DI), the Jenkins activity survey (JAS), the Framingham type A scale, and the Bortner rating scale. The SI was originally developed by Friedman and Rosenman for their studies of middle-class employed men. The classification of men as type A (A_1 or A_2), type B, or type X (equally A and B) was based on self-reports of type A behaviour during the interview (competitive, doing things quickly, multiphasic thinking), speech stylistics (such as speed of answering questions, loud voice, or explosive speech), and behavioural mannerisms (interruptions to interviewer's questions, speech hurrying, or one-word responses).[3] The SI has been considered the standard measurement technique for men. The other self-reported pencil and paper questionnaires have a modest agreement with the SI (60–70%) classification in men, and contain different questions in a variety of response formats, for example, JAS (50 items), Framingham (10 items), and Bortner (14 items).

The validity of the SI for women has received little attention to date and requires future investigation. Several concerns should be raised with the structured interview assessment technique for women. Firstly, the type A behaviour assessed in the SI may be socially acceptable for men but not for women (for example, loud voice and competitiveness). Thus, women would be less likely to exhibit these mannerisms than men. Likewise, some behaviours used to classify men as type A—for example, interruptions—may be far more common and part of the social norm for women. Secondly, many questions used in the SI are work-oriented, making their content inappropriate for eliciting type A responses among housewives. Questions on competition with children in games may elicit different responses from mothers than from single women. Alternatively, the SI is a much more sensitive measure for eliciting the stylistics and behavioural mannerisms that cannot be revealed in pencil and paper questionnaires. Response bias for content is also less likely to occur with the interview.

In order to answer these questions, several comparisons are required. The weighting of voice stylistics used in the SI for assessing men as type A should be compared with comparable stylistics for women. In addition, the concordance of pencil and paper measures with the SI should help in determining the agreement of reported content across instruments. Finally, the risks of developing CHD should be compared for the SI and self-assessment questionnaires to examine their respective predictive validities.

To date, seven studies have administered the SI among non-clinical population-based groups of women (see Table 7.1).[4-10] The agreement between various self-reported type A questionnaires with the SI has been disappointing. In a comprehensive validation study of the SI in women, Anderson and Waldron[8] reported a 54% agreement between the SI and JAS assessment of type A behaviour in 88 women

67

Table 7.1 Distribution of type A behaviour among women in various population groups. SI = structured interview, JAS = Jenkins activity survey

Investigator/year	Site and study	Sample characteristics	Type A measure	Percentage of mean scores
Rosenman, Friedman 1961[4]	California employed women	257 women, aged 30–59	lay nomination and SI	49% type A
Smyth et al 1978[5]	Chicago inner city ghetto	31 black women, aged 20–52	SI	45% type A
Haynes et al 1980[6]	Massachusetts Framingham Heart Study	77 white women, aged 55–64	SI	51% type A
MacDougal et al 1981[7]	Florida, psychology students	60 women, aged 18–27	SI	48–55% type A
Anderson, Waldron 1983[8]	Pennsylvania neighbourhood sample and Protestant church members	88 white women, aged 40–59	SI	70% type A
Meininger, Zyzanski 1983[9]	Northeastern US hospital employees	149 white women, aged 30–42	SI	44% type A
Moss 1984[10]	Washtenaw County, Michigan Health Survey	912 men and women aged 17–34	SI	43% type A
Shekelle et al 1976[11]	Chicago, Chicago Heart Association Detection Project	876 white women, aged 25–64	JAS	25–44: -2.2 45–64: -4.7 mean
Waldron et al 1977[12]	Chicago, Chicago Heart Association Detection Project in Industry	1149 white women, 266 black women, aged 18–64	JAS	-4.3 mean
Glass 1977[13]	Austin, University of Texas undergraduates	100–150 women, age not stated	JAS	About 50% type A
Waldron 1978[14]	Pennsylvania neighbourhood sample and Protestant church members	92 white women, aged 40–59	JAS	Full-time employment, -2.7 mean; part-time employment, -5.8 mean
Waldron et al 1980[15]	Philadelphia, University of Pennsylvania undergraduate students	28 women, age not stated	JAS	0.5 mean
McCranie et al 1981[16]	Georgia, medical students	17 women, age not stated	JAS	47% type A
Loewenstine, Paludi 1982[17]	Psychology students	65 women, age not stated	JAS	7.3 mean

Table 7.1 (*cont.*)

Investigator/year	Site and study	Sample characteristics	Type A measure	Percentage of mean scores
Morell, Katkin 1982[18]	Buffalo, State University of New York employees and their wives	299 women, age not stated	JAS	Professionals had significantly higher scores than homemakers
Lawler et al 1983[19]	Tennessee, professional and executive women, and housewives	41 women, aged 25–55	JAS	Employed As: 10.9 mean; unemployed As: 7.6 mean; unemployed Bs: -7.9 or 73% A
Davidson et al 1980[20]	England, managers and administrators in Women's Who's Who	148 women, aged 21–60	Bortner	59% type A
Bernet et al 1982[21]	France, Marseilles Council employees	768 women, aged 21–65	Bortner	21–39: 10% 40–65: 25% type A
Haynes et al 1978[22]	Massachusetts, Framingham Heart Study	1011 white women, aged 45–77	Framingham type A	Working women: 57% housewives: 41% type A

aged 40–59. When the type Xs were excluded, the concordance rate was 47%. Likewise, among 77 Framingham cohort women aged 55–64, the agreement rates were 5% overall and 55% excluding Xs.[11] Meininger and Zyzanski reported agreement rates of 45.6% for the Framingham scale and 49% for the JAS in 149 white women in the northeastern US.[9] These agreement rates are lower than the 67–73% agreement with the SI observed among men for the JAS[23, 24] and the 60% agreement among men for the Framingham scale.[6] The poor concordance rates suggest that with women the SI ratings may give more weight to speech stylistics than to content. Further analysis of the Anderson and Waldron sample suggested that the JAS type A scores were more closely related to the content of interview responses and that behaviour and the content of responses may not be related.

Of additional interest is the extent to which the stylistics used to identify type A men are similar in the assessment of type A women. Again, the Framingham and Pennsylvania studies provided some basis for comparison. Table 7.2 summarises preliminary results from voice coding of the SI which was completed under the direction of Jacobs from the University of Minnesota. Tapes from 77 Framingham Heart Study women and from a subsample of 98 men in the original Western Collaborative Group Study (WCGS) were analysed using published procedures.[25] As can be seen, the four most significant predictors of a type A classification in men were the number of explosive words (that is, words that have an explosive quality), volume of voice (1–4, soft to loud) based on code ratings, speed of answering or responding to questions (1–5, slow to fast), and overall speed of speech (1–5, slow to fast). These four variables accounted for 35% of the variance in type A scores for men.

Among women a somewhat different pattern emerged, with overall speed being the only comparable significant stylistic. The most significant factor in women was delay latency—that is, the time (in tenths of seconds) between a stammer, on one of the type A questions and the response of the interviewee, and uneven speed in answering—that is, degree to which last words of a sentence are spoken at a faster rate than first words (1–3, infrequent to often). These variables accounted for 39% of the variance in type A scores. It is interesting that interruptions were the fourth most important predictor in women and the twelfth or next to last most important predictor in men.

Table 7.2 Preliminary results from voice-coding analysis. Variables most predictive of type A-B behaviour measured by interviews.

Western Collaborative Group Study men (n=98)		Framingham Heart Study Women (n=77)	
Stylistic	F-test	Stylistic	F-test
Explosive words	8.02*	Delay latency	12.58*
Volume of voice	7.49*	Speed	9.16*
Speed of answering	7.37*	Uneven speed	6.59*
Speed	4.76*		
(Multiple R=0.59,	R2=0.35)	(Multiple R=0.62,	R2=0.39)
Delay latency	3.07	Interruptions	2.64
Repeated words	1.77	Explosive words	2.15
Uneven speed	1.23	Speed of answering	1.63
Volume changes	1.07	Volume changes	1.17
Length of interview	0.82	Volume of voice	0.55
Speed change	0.70	Clipped words	0.42
Clipped words	0.56	Speed change	0.36
Interruptions	0.42	Repeated words	0.31
Sighs	0.33	Length of interview	0.22
		Sighs	0.20

*p<0.05
Note: The volume of voice was positively correlated with explosive words in men (r=0.26), but was negatively correlated with explosive words in women (r=0.21).

Anderson and Waldron[8] reported similar findings in their voice analysis of the SI, with rate of speaking (r=0.67), word emphasis (r=0.55), hurried motor pace (r=0.49), and average response latency (r=0.38) as the four strongest correlates of the SI rating. Thus, the importance of certain voice stylistics in the SI assessment are different for men and women. In particular, voice stylistics such as volume of voice appear to be more important predictors of the SI assessment among men, while speed and delay latency are important predictors of the type A behaviour rating among women. Further developmental work of this nature is required to evaluate adequately the robustness of the SI for use among women.

Given these limitations for the structured interview assessment of type A behaviour, it is interesting to note in Table 7.1 the remarkable similarity in the distribution of type A behaviour among women in different populations through-out the US. Five of six studies using the SI reported similar percentages of women classified as type A, 44–55%.[4 7.9] The JAS scores among women were generally positive and higher among students, professional women, and employed

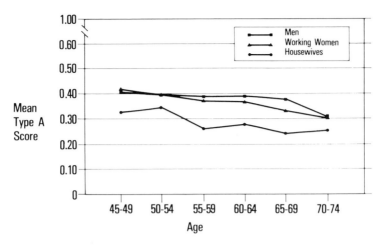

Fig. 7.1 Framingham type A scores by age, sex, and employment status.

women. In Framingham, for example, although the scale was dichotomised at the median to distinguish type A from type B women, at each age (45–54, 55–64 and 65–74) 16% more working women than housewives were classified as type A (57% vs 41%).[22]   The relationship between type A behaviour and age is complex and inconsistent across studies. Using data from the Chicago Heart Association Detection Project in Industry, Waldron et al[12] reported a rise in JAS type A scores to a peak at about ages 30–35, followed by a steady decline thereafter. Figure 7.1 illustrates a steady decline in Framingham type A scores with age after 45 years for working women, housewives, and men. As in the Chicago Project,[12] no sex differences were observed among the employed people in Framingham. Likewise, men and working women in Framingham had almost identical mean scores, but housewives had significantly lower mean type A scores in the Framingham study (0.29) than working women (0.37).[22]

In summary, based on current knowledge one must conclude that the best assessment technique for type A behaviour in women has yet to be determined. In addition, and of some surprise, is the apparent lack of a sex difference in type A behaviour among employed people. This suggests that women who enter the work force may be expected to assume the hard-driving, time-urgent behaviours of their male counterparts in order to succeed, feel comfortable with, or cope with the Westernised system of employment. Alternatively, type A women could self-select to enter the work place. As more women enter the work force, however, the effect of self-selection of type A could disappear as the proportion of women in the labour force reaches 70% or more—that is, exceeds the proportion of women who are type A in the population.

PROSPECTIVE, CASE-CONTROL, AND HIGH-RISK INDIVIDUAL STUDIES

Prospective studies
The first and, to date, only prospective study designed to test the coronary risk

associated with type A behaviour in women was the Framingham Heart Study.[6,22,26,27] Between 1965 and 1967, 1822 men and women aged 45–77 years were given an extensive psychosocial questionnaire. The questionnaire encompassed measures of behaviour types (for example, type A behaviour) as well as situational stress (for example, work overload), anger-coping styles (for example, anger-in, anger-out, anger-discuss), somatic strains (for example, anxiety), and sociodemographic characteristics (for example, marital status, children, occupation). The 725 men and 949 women who were free of CHD at their eighth or ninth biennial examination were followed for the development of CHD over 8 and 10 year periods.[6,27]

These studies showed that type A behaviour, as defined by a ten-item questionnaire on time-urgency and competitiveness, was significantly related to the 8 year incidence of CHD among women and men—and particularly men employed in white-collar jobs. The relative risks were 2.1, 1.8, and 2.9 for people aged 45–64 years in these three groups (women, men, men in white-collar jobs) and were significant when controlled for the standard coronary risk factors. Although the white-collar work environment seemed to increase the risk of CHD for type A men, type A risks were not higher among women working outside the home. That is, the relative risk for CHD among type A compared with type B working women was 1.6 whereas the comparable relative risk among housewives was 2.9, (p < 0.05). Since very few Framingham women were employed in white-collar jobs (primarily as teachers, nurses, or librarians), the the synergistic effect of high-pressure work environments and type A behaviour observed among men could not be tested among women.

At the 10 year follow-up, the relationship of type A behaviour to various manifestations of CHD was explored further.[27] Among both men and women, type A behaviour was associated only with coronary disease in which symptoms of angina pectoris were presented—that is, when the subject reported symptoms of substernal discomfort of short duration (less than 15 minutes) directly related to exertion or excitement and relieved by rest or nitroglycerin. In that study, angina pectoris only (APO) was designated when angina was the initial and only manifestation of CHD during the 10 year period. Angina pectoris (AP) included all cases of angina, regardless of the development of other clinical manifestations of CHD such as myocardial infarction (MI), coronary insufficiency syndrome, or CHD death (sudden and non-sudden). Complicated MI occurred when an MI was associated with angina, either before, after, or at the same examination as the MI diagnosis.

At the 10 year follow-up, the relative risks of developing all forms of CHD were 1.4 for all men, 2.4 for white-collar men, and 2.0 for women, for those aged 45–64 years. As seen in Figure 7.2, the relative risk for CHD among type A as compared with type B working women was 1.6 (p=0.17), whereas the comparable relative risk for housewives was 2.4 (p=0.02). Among men aged 45–64 years, type A behaviour was also associated with APO, AP, and complicated MI, with type As incurring about twice the risk of developing each diagnosis over the subsequent 10 years as the type Bs (relative risks of 1.8, 1.9, and 2.6, respectively), (p<0.05). Likewise, among women of comparable age, type A behaviour was significantly associated only with the development of APO and AP, with relative risks of 2.6 and 2.2, respectively

72

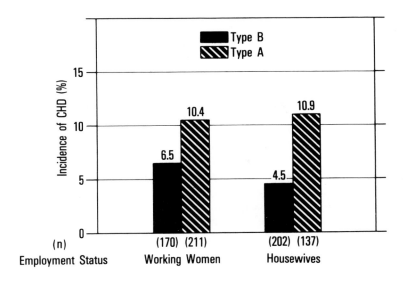

Fig. 7.2 Ten-year incidence of CHD among women aged 45–64 years by employment status and Framingham type A behaviour.

(p=0.02). Surprisingly, among both men and women, type As and type Bs had almost identical rates of MIs which presented with no other manifestation of CHD.

Three important lessons may be learnt from the Framingham study about the association between type A behaviour and employment, status, and CHD. Firstly, the relative risks of developing CHD for type A women were higher among housewives than working women. This does not imply, however, that type A

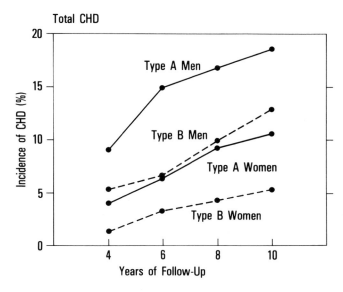

Fig. 7.3 Incidence of CHD among men and women aged 45–64 years by type A behaviour after 4, 6, 8, and 10 years follow-up.

working women are not at additional coronary risk, since type A working women had similar coronary rates to type A housewives (10.4 vs 10.9%). Given these rates, the lower relative risks among working women were due to higher rates among type B working women than among type B housewives (Fig. 7.2). The results suggest that working in the home does not protect type A women from higher rates of coronary disease. Alternatively, the results also suggest that working outside the home may not necessarily be accompanied by excess coronary risk for type A women.

Secondly, if employed women follow the pattern or experience of executive men, one must be concerned about the excessive risk of CHD among white-collar men (relative risk=2.9 at the 8 year follow-up). These men were employed as professionals, managers, and businessmen. Women must be cautioned to avoid the behaviours, time-pressured situations, or executive stress of white-collar jobs in which men have predominated for decades.

Finally, despite the excessive risks among type A women in Framingham, their rates did not approach the rates for type A men (Fig. 7.3). In fact, type A women had almost identical rates of CHD to type B, not type A, men. This finding may be explained by at least four phenomena:

1. protective hormonal factors inherent in women or
2. by the fact that women have different work pressures from type A men, or
3. that women have some protective coping mechanisms for stress not used by men, or
4. that type A women leave the work force sooner, change their behaviour sooner, and seek medical care sooner than men when afflicted with anginal chest pain.

From a clinical viewpoint, two additional questions arise from the Framingham findings. Firstly, since type A behaviour in women was associated with angina-related coronary disease, do the results reflect true coronary disease and atherosclerosis or just the propensity to report chest pain? Secondly, how many more coronary cases can we identify over and above the standard risk factors by knowing a woman's behaviour type?

In response to the question, the diagnosis of angina used in Framingham is different from the more commonly used methods in epidemiology. In Framingham, angina pectoris was diagnosed when symptoms were experienced of substantial discomfort of less than 15 minutes, distinctly related to exertion or excitement, and relieved by rest or nitroglycerin. This diagnosis was confirmed only after a review from a panel of clinical investigators. This method of assessing angina is thought to be more valid than the self-reported questionnaires such as the Rose questionnaire for angina.

Although women presenting with angina have a better prognosis than men in Framingham, Kannel and Feinleib[28] have shown that 40% of all women aged 60–69 who had uncomplicated angina died within 8 years. This rate was comparable to the mortality among men aged 50–69. For younger women, aged 50–59, the 8 year mortality was substantially lower, at 15%. Thus, the occurrence of angina in women has fairly serious consequences, despite the common assumption that the diagnosis of angina is a 'soft-endpoint'. Studies examining type A behaviour and the severity of atherosclerosis will be summarised later in this chapter.

74

Figure 7.4 shows the percentage of coronary cases after 8 years' follow-up according to quintiles of risk determined by either the standard coronary risk factors alone or by the standard risk factors plus type A behaviour and anger-discuss. The anger-discuss variable was also a significant predictor of CHD among women, in that women who did not usually discuss their anger were significantly more likely to develop CHD than those who did. In Figure 7.4, the population has been stratified into five risk groups according to scores from a logistic regression equation, which included the standard coronary risk factors of systolic blood pressure, serum cholesterol, cigarette smoking, and age. The upper quintile of risk groups, then, are likely to have several of the noted coronary risk factors. For women aged 45–64, 48% of the incident coronary cases were found in the upper quintile of risk when only the standard risk factors were used in the scoring. When the behavioural variables were included in the scoring, 63% of the coronary cases were located in the upper quintile of risk. In women, therefore, we were able to identify 16% more coronary cases in the high-risk group by taking type A behaviour and anger-coping style into account.

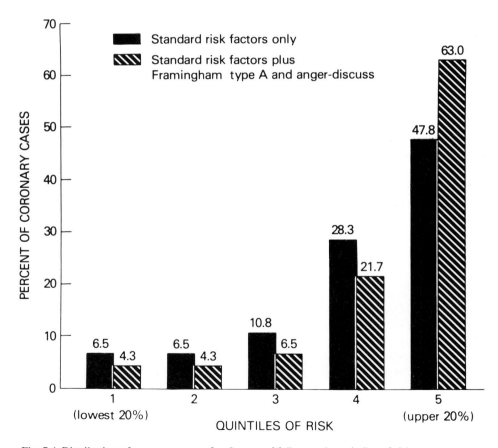

Fig. 7.4 Distribution of coronary cases after 8 years of follow-up by quintiles of risk among women aged 45–64 years.

Case-control, prevalence, and high-risk studies

The study of coronary risk factors among women has received little attention compared with studies among men. Only five investigators [4,11,22,29,30] have assessed type A behaviours among women in regard to the presence of coronary disease. These studies are summarised in Table 7.3.

In 1961, Rosenman and Friedman[4] found the prevalence of CHD about four times greater among extreme type A than among extreme type B women. In a case-control study, Kenigsberg et al[30] found that women with CHD scored significantly

Table 7.3 Review of case-control, prevalence, and coronary angiography studies in women.

Investi-gator/year	Population studied	Type A measure	Disease measure	Findings
Rosenman, Friedman 1961[4]	257 women in California, aged 30–59	Lay nomina-tion and SI	% clinical coronary disease	*Pattern A:* Premen 9.8 Postmen 37.2 *Pattern B:* Premen 2.7 Postmen 9.0 Difference in % CHD
Bengtsson et al 1973[29]	42 women with MI, 68 population controls, mean age 54	Cesarcic-Markes Person-ality Schedule aggression, neurotic self-assertiveness	MI cases vs population controls	*Aggression* MI—4.9 Ref—3.7 £ < 0.05 *Neuroticism* MI—1146.3 Ref—128.6 p< 0.05
Kenigsberg et al 1974[30]	21 inpatients at Bridgeport Hospital, aged 22–64	JAS	CHD cases vs injury and surgery controls	Cases: 1.30 mean Controls: 0.06 on JAS dif-ference sig-nificant
Haynes et al 1978[26]	Framingham, Massachusetts 1011 white women, aged 45–77	Framingham type A	CHD prevalence rates	*Type A:* 45–54 0.5% 55–64 2.4% 64+ 9.3% *Type B:* 45–54 4.0% 55–64 7.7% 65+ 20.0% p < 0.01 for continuous measure
Blumenthal et al 1978[31]	62 Duke Uni-versity Hos-pital women, aged 15–69	SI JAS	TOTCI Atheroscle-rosis score (0–12)	Mean TOTCI for women= 1.5; SI, not JAS related to TOTCI; p < 0.001
Frank et al 1978[32]	23 women at Columbia Pres Med Ctr, aged 29–65	SI	Number of arteries occluded > 50%	Male sex correlated with disease severity, r280.29, SI related to occlusion, p> 0.05

Table 7.3 *(contd.)*

Investigator/year	Population studied	Type A measure	Disease measure	Findings
Silver et al 1980[33]	78 women at Boston University Medical Ctr, aged 25–68	JAS	CAD patients vs valve and other diseases CAD vs valve	Job involvement of JAS greater in women patients (-10.7 vs -6.1, resp, p280.057)
Williams et al 1980[34]	117 women at Duke University Medical Ctr, age not stated	SI	$\geqslant 75\%$ stenosis in one or more arteries non-hostile	3.6 relative risk type A hostile vs non type A
Bass and Wade 1982[35]	32 women at Kings College Hospital	Bortner	0, $< 50\%$ in one + vessel, and $> 50\%$ stenosis in 1+ vessel	No association, 028 168.3 mean, $< 50\%28$ 174.6, $> 50\%$ 168.8
Abbott 1983[36]	35 women at University of Pittsburgh Hospital, aged 26–58	Framingham type A	Number of vessels with $> 50\%$ occlusion, CAD vs no CAD	r280.294 phi correlation coefficient, p280.04
Pearson 1983[37]	120 white, 12 black women at Johns Hopkins Hospital	Bortner	Number of vessels with $> 50\%$ narrowing, CAD vs no CAD	No association, WW: cases— 185.7 mean controls— 182.0; BW: 171.5 controls— 185.4
Haynes et al 1984[38]	299 white women at Duke University Hospital, aged 35–74	SI, Framingham type A, JAS	$> 50\%$ occlusion in one or more arteries	Significant association of SI with CAD in women 35–44 only; Type A: 36.4% Type B: 7.7% p=0.008 No significant association with Framingham or JAS

higher than non-cardiovascular hospital controls on the JAS type A scale. The Swedish study by Bengtsson et al[29] is one of the most comprehensive studies of risk factors for myocardial infarction and angina pectoris in women. In that study women with MI scored significantly higher on aggression and neurotic self-assertiveness scales than the population-based controls, the calculations being made from scores of achievement, guilt feelings, deference of status, and aggression. None of the personality traits scored significantly higher in the AP group than in the reference group. However, angina was assessed by the Rose questionnaire. Since neuroticism has been shown to correlate highly with the Framingham type A scale in men (r=0.45),[39] the Swedish results are more or less consistent with the Framingham prevalence results. The lack of significant associations with angina in the Swedish study may be explained by the limited number of angina cases,[29] and/or the less reliable method of assessing angina in women, that is, Rose questionnaire. A key question raised by the Swedish study is the possibility that neuroticism, or self-esteem, along with aggressiveness may be important components of coronary-prone behaviour among women.

In the Framingham Prevalence Study,[22] type A women were significantly more likely to have prevalent coronary disease than type B women, at all ages and in all employment groups. Risk ratios of coronary prevalence rates among type A compared with type B working women ranged from 2.6, 3.2, and 4.2 for age groups 45-54, 55-64, and 65+. Rate ratios for type A housewives were 3.1, 1.4 for age groups 55-64 and 65+, with rates of 0 and 5.9% for type B and type A housewives, aged 45-54. Hence the relative risks rose with age for type A as compared with type B working women, and declined with age among housewives. As with the incidence data, the associations were strongest for APO and AP—that is, diagnosis related to angina.

In Table 7.3, eight angiography studies comparing type A behaviour with the degree of atherosclerosis are reviewed. Almost all the women referred to angiography had reported anginal pain. Six of the eight studies show a positive association between the SI, JAS, or Framingham scale and the degree of atherosclerosis. Three of the six positive findings, however, are from the Duke University Medical Center sample.[32,38,39] No associations are observed between the Bortner measure of type A behaviour and coronary stenosis in the two studies which used this scale.[35,37] In addition, there is some suggestion that the type A-atherosclerosis association in women may be related to job involvement behaviour[33] or to hostile behaviour.[34]

In summary, the case-control, prevalence, and angiography studies examining type A behaviour and coronary disease in women have shown positive associations. Although the Framingham data suggested that the type A association operated through the presence of angina pectoris, the angiography studies show an association with atherosclerosis severity in the presence of severe angina. These studies provide some evidence that there is a biological rather than psychological mechanism through which type A is linked to the development of CHD and atherosclerosis.

TYPE A BEHAVIOUR, STANDARD CORONARY RISK FACTORS, AND PHYSIOLOGICAL REACTIVITY

The accumulated evidence presented so far suggests that type A behaviour is a significant risk factor for the development of CHD and atherosclerosis in women. The biological mechanism by which type A exerts a pathogenic effect on the cardiovascular system is of crucial importance. At least two schools of thought have led to investigations in this area. The first approach, which may be called the 'static' model, includes the examination of biological variables that might be correlated with type A behaviour, and which are also risk factors for the development of CHD.

Here, resting levels of the standard coronary risk factors of systolic and diastolic blood pressure, serum cholesterol, cigarette smoking, and obesity have been tested for their association with type A behaviour. If there is a positive correlation, some or all of the association between type A behaviour and CHD might be explained.

Table 7.4 Review of type A behaviour, standard coronary risk factors, and physiological reactivity studies.

Investigator/year	Population studied	Type A measure	Findings
Static measures:			
Shekelle et al 1976[11]	876 women in Chicago Heart Assoc. Detection Project in Industry	JAS	Cigarette smoking significantly associated (+) with JAS in younger working women aged 25–44, hypertension significantly associated with JAS in older working women, aged 45–64. No association for women with probability of developing CHD estimated by Framingham equation.
Haynes et al 1978[26]	1011 white Framingham Heart Study women, aged 45–77	Framingham type A	No significant correlations with SBP, DBP, serum cholesterol, or cigarette smoking for all women. For white-collar women 65, r28.25 with serum cholesterol
Smyth et al 1978[5]	33 black Chicago inner city women, aged 20–62	SI	Type As did not have significantly higher mean systolic, diastolic or mean arterial pressure
Waldron et at 1980[15]	28 University of Pennsylvania women students	JAS	Type A scores were not correlated with average blood pressures, heart rate, or obesity.
McCranie et al 1981[16]	17 women medical students in Georgia	JAS	Type A compared with type B women had higher total cholesterol, higher LDL, lower HDL, and higher systolic and diastolic blood pressures.
Change measures:			
Manuck et al 1978[40]	26 women psychology students	Sales Type A	No differences were observed between type A and type B women in systolic blood pressure after taking a series of tests.

Table 7.4 (*contd*).

Investigator/year	Population studied	Type A measure	Findings
MacDougall et al 1981[7]	60 women Eckerd College students	SI JAS	SI type A behaviour associated with increases in systolic blood pressure during interview and American History quiz, but not re- action time task. JAS and Framingham type A not correlate with HR or blood pressure change.
Lawler et al 1983[19]	41 women professionals, aged 25–55	JAS	Type A women showed higher heart rates and larger increases in systolic and dia- stolic pressures in response to maths tests and puzzle- solving. Unemployed As had greatest blood pressure responses.
Lane et al 1984[41]	29 Duke University women students	JAS	None of the JAS scales, A-B, Spd-Imp Hrd-Cmp were related to heart rate, SBP, DBP, Forearm blood flow vascular resis- tance in response to mental arithmetic or task performance.
Frankenhaeuser et al 1980[42]	24 female university students, aged 18–27	JAS	Type A women did not differ significantly from type Bs in adrenaline or non- adrenaline excretion, heart rate, or cortisol excretion in response to a choice reaction task.

Table 7.4 summarises results from studies which have examined the correlations between type A behaviour and the standard risk factors for CHD. As a whole, type As do not appear to have higher levels of blood pressure, serum cholesterol, cigarette smoking, or obesity than type Bs. The correlations between these measures are low and in most cases not significant.

These findings do not imply, however, that type A behaviour does not combine with the standard risk factors either in an additive or synergistic fashion in the development of CHD. As can be seen in Figure 7.5, a synergistic relationship did exist in the Framingham cohort women between type A behaviour and the standard coronary risk factors in the development of CHD.[27] The curves show the expected or smoothed 10 year incidence rates of CHD among type A and type B women according to their risk of developing CHD based on age, systolic blood pressure,

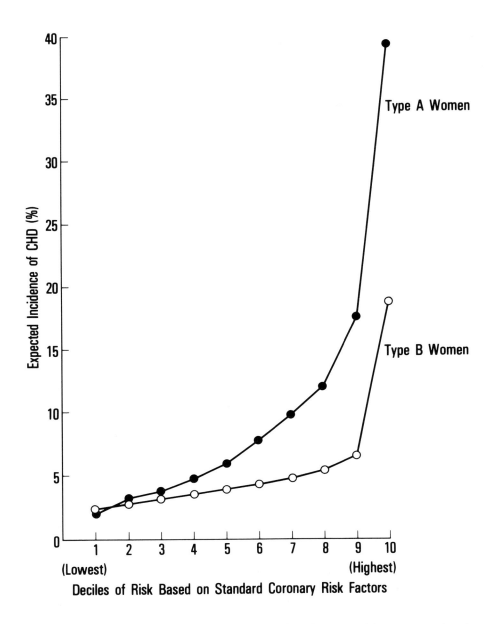

Fig. 7.5 Expected 10 year incidence rates of CHD by deciles of coronary risk among type A and type B women aged 45–64 years.

serum cholesterol, and cigarette smoking. As the levels of the standard coronary risk factors increased for women, the difference between CHD rates for type As and type Bs also increased. In fact, the relative risk (type A/ type B) for CHD incidence among women was significant only in the top decile of risk, based on the standard coronary risk factors (relative risk=2.1 with confidence limits 1.0–4.5).

A second approach to this research, which may be called the 'dynamic' model, has argued that as type As chronically respond to stimulating environmental challenges, their sympathetic nervous system and adrenomedullary activity is increased, leading them to a heightened physiological reactivity compared with type Bs. It has been suggested that this reactivity explains the excess rates of CHD among type A women. These investigations have examined both resting measures of sympathetic nervous system activity, as well as change after exposure to a variety of laboratory stressors or stimuli. Biological measures such as heart rate, blood pressure, skin resistance, plasma and urinary catecholamines, and cortisol have most often been examined. Table 7.4 summarises the results from these studies among women.

On the whole, the results from five studies on this subject have been disappointing. Of particular note is the lack of association in studies which have used reaction time tests as the environmental challenge in laboratory experiments.[40-42] The two positive studies by MacDougall et al[7] and Lawler et al[19] observed significant differences in blood pressure (systolic and diastolic) change among type A and type B women during academic exercises such as history quizzes, mathematics tests, and puzzle solving. Because Frankenhaeuser[43] observed that women did not show the same rises in adrenaline to various testing challenges as men, it was suggested that the explanation for the sex difference in reactivity might be related to type A behaviour. Unfortunately, type A behaviour in women, per se, did not explain the significant sex differences in adrenaline rise induced by an achievement choice-reaction-time test in the laboratory.[42]

The Lawler study[19] deserves further comment because it was the first study to examine psychophysiological responses to stress in adult working and homemaking women. In a predominately type A (73%) group of adult women (aged 25–55), heart rate and systolic, and diastolic blood pressures rose in response to mathematical and Raven's tests. The unemployed type A group responded the greatest to these tests with regard to blood pressure change, and the employed type As responded with the greatest change in heart rate. Six of the nine unemployed type As said they would prefer to work rather than stay at home. Lawler et al[19] cautioned that one might expect to see higher rates of CHD incidence in the future, because many employed women are 'as type A as men' in their reactivity to stress.

From an epidemiological viewpoint, the sample sizes, age range, and occupation groups in all published studies to date are limited in their ability to draw reliable conclusions. Lawler et al[19] have paved the way for research in this area, which it is hoped will include more diverse populations of women in a variety of settings. Researchers must use comparable or identical instruments in laboratory experiments so that differences between studies are not due solely to the use of different experimental challenges. Recommendations for the best choice of instruments for psychophysiological studies among women would be welcomed from scientists doing research on this subject.

EMPLOYMENT, OCCUPATION, AND FAMILY RESPONSIBILITIES

The evidence accumulated to date suggests that type A behaviour is a significant risk factor for CHD. Because this behaviour is far more predominant in women who work outside the home, and among high occupational status groups, concern has been raised that employment, per se, may lead to higher coronary incidence rates and coronary risk factor levels.

The Framingham study was the first prospective study to examine the effect of employment, occupation, family responsibilities, and behaviour on CHD incidence rates in women.[44] After 8 years' follow-up, no significant differences were observed between working women and housewives (7.8 vs 5.4%, respectively). Nevertheless, CHD rates were twice as great among women holding clerical jobs (10.6%) as among housewives or other occupation groups. White-collar women, employed primarily as teachers, nurses, or librarians had the lowest incidence rates of any occupational group studied (5.2%).

The work environment, as well as the family environment, of the clerical worker contributes to her excess coronary risk. One out of 5 (or 21.3%) of these workers developed coronary disease if they had raised children and were married to blue-collar husbands. In contrast, single clerical working women had the lowest risks of developing CHD (3.7%). In addition to family responsibilities, the most significant risk factors for CHD in this group of women were not discussing one's anger and having a non-supportive boss. These findings have been confirmed in both the 8 and 10 year follow-up studies.[44,45]

The Framingham findings suggested that clerical workers may experience severe occupational stress, including a lack of autonomy and control over the work environment, underuse of skills, and lack of recognition of their accomplishments. The common thread linking clerical work and type A behaviour as risk factors for CHD is the issue of control. The clerical job has been classified as having high demands and low control, job characteristics which have been shown by Karasek and others to be associated with an excess risk of coronary disease in men.[46] Likewise, the Framingham type A scale and the JAS speed and impatience scale have been shown to be negatively correlated with control ($r=-0.24$ and -0.20, respectively).[47,48] Since the Framingham type A and JAS speed and impatience scales are highly intercorrelated ($r=0.50$ or greater),[6,49] their association with control scales is not surprising.

In one instance (clerical work), lack of control is created by work environment. In the other case (type A behaviour), lack of control may result from either self-perception or from the work environment.

Several investigators have shown that lack of control at work is related to systolic and diastolic blood pressure, excretion of catecholamines, hypertension, and prevalence and incidence of cardiovascular disease and mortality in men.[46,50-54] To explore this factor in more depth, a re-analysis of the Framingham data has recently been completed by LaCroix and Haynes.[55] Working women were stratified into four control groups: low-high, high-low, low-low, and high-high. The 10 year incidence of CHD in these groups were 2.4, 5.6, 13.6, and 31.3% respectively. Overall, clerical workers with high demands and low control were 5.2 times ($p \pi 0.5$) more likely to develop CHD than the other three groups combined, after controlling for the standard coronary risk factors.[55]

This effect of control on the risk of coronary disease in women merits further attention, particularly working women who generally hold jobs with low control and decision-making.

FUTURE RESEARCH

The accumulated published work on women and heart disease reviewed in this paper was limited by the few studies that have focused on women. The following research questions are posed to close the gender gap which exists in our current knowledge about type A behaviour, employment status, and CHD in women. Some research questions suggested by Haw[56] in a comprehensive review of publication on women, work and stress were considered.

1. What aspects of the job environment are responsible for the excess rates among high-risk occupations in women, for example clerical work? Specifically, what effect does underutilisation of skills, lack of autonomy and control, lack of recognition for accomplishment, presence of challenges, and excessive hours have on incidence rates of CHD?

2. What are the best and worst coping styles for women in adapting to work-related stress? Is anger expression, anger suppression, or some other coping mechanism more beneficial to one's cardiovascular health?

3. What effect do multiple roles and family responsibilities (employed woman, wife, and mother) have on CHD rates in type A women? Do husbands' attitudes and shared household responsibilities enhance or protect the type A working woman from the development of CHD?

4. What is the physiological process, objectively measured in the laboratory or, preferably, in the work place, through which high-risk occupations or behaviours manifest themselves in CHD?

In closing, it is hoped that future studies will examine some of the issues raised surrounding the cardiovascular health of employed women. It would be an historical error to ignore the natural experiment which is taking place in America today, that is, a situation where half of the women work inside the home and half of the women work outside the home. Knowledge concerning the effect of work on the pathogenesis of coronary disease in women may also provide valuable insights into the effect of work on the cardiovascular health of men.

REFERENCES

[1]The Review Panel on Coronary-Prone Behavior and Coronary Heart Disease. Coronary-prone behavior and coronary heart disease: a critical review. Circulation 1981; 63: 1199–215.

[2]Friedman M, Rosenman RH. Type A behavior pattern: Its association with coronary heart diseases. Ann Clin Res 1971; 3: 300–12.

[3]Rosenman RH. The interview method of assessment of the coronary-prone behavior pattern. In: Dembroski TM, Weiss SM, Shields JL, Haynes SG, Feinleib M, eds. Coronary-prone behavior. New York, Heidelberg, Berlin: Springer, 1978: 55–70.

[4]Rosenman RH, Friedman M. Association of specific behavior pattern in women with blood and cardiovascular findings. Circulation 1961; 24: 1173–84.

[5]Smyth K, Call J, Hansell S, Sparacino J, Strodtbeck FL. Type A behavior pattern and hypertension among inner-city black women. Nursing Res 1978; 27: 30–5.

[6]Haynes SG, Feinleib M, Kannel WB. The relationship of psychosocial factors to coronary heart disease in the Framingham Study III. Eight-year incidence of coronary heart disease. Am J Epidemiol 1980; 3: 37–58.

[7]MacDougall JM, Dembroski TM, Krantz DS. Effects of types of challenge on pressor and heart rate responses in Type A and Type B women. Psychophysiology 1981; 18: 1–9.

[8] Anderson JR, Waldron I. Behavioral and content components of the structured interview assessment of the Type A behavior pattern in women. J Behav Med 1983; 6: 123–34.

[9] Meininger J. Zyzanski S. The validity of Type A behavior scales for employed women. Am J Epidemiol 1983; 118: 424 (abstract).

[10] Moss GE. The sociodemographic distribution of Type A behavior in population sample. Psychosom Med 1984; 46: 85–6.

[11] ShekellerRB, Schoenberger JA, Stamler J. Correlates of the JAS Type A behavior pattern score. J Chronic Dis 1976; 29: 381–94.

[12] Waldron I, Zyzanski S, Shekelle RB, Jenkins CD, Tannebaum S. The coronary-prone behavior pattern in employed men and women. J Human Stress 1977; 3: 2–18.

[13] Glass DC, Behavior patterns, stress, and coronary disease. Hillsdale, New Jersey: Lawrence Erlbaum Assoc, 1977.

[14] Waldron I. The coronary-prone behavior pattern, blood pressure, employment and socio-economic status in women. J Psychosom Res 1978; 22: 79–87.

[15] Waldron I, Hickey A, McPherson C et al. Type A behavior pattern: relationship to variation in blood pressure, parental characteristics, and academic and social activities of students. J Human Stress 1980; 6: 16–27.

[16] McCranie EW, Simpson ME, Stevens JS. Type A behavior, field dependence, and serum lipids. Psychosom Med 1981; 43: 107.

[17] Loewenstine HV, Paludi MA. Women's type A/B behavior patterns and fear of success. Percept Mot Skills 1982; 54: 891–4.

[18] Morell MA, Katkin ES. Jenkins Activity Survey scores among women of different occupations. J Consult Clin Psychol 1982; 4: 588–9.

[19] Lawler KA, Rixse A, Allen MT. Type A behavior and psychophysiological response in adult women. Psychophysiology 1983; 20: 343–50.

[20] Davidson MJ, Cooper CL, Chamberlain D. Type A coronary-prone behavior and stress in senior female managers and administrators. J Occup Med 1980; 22: 801–5.

[21] Bernet A, Drivet-Perrin J, Blanc MM, Ebagosti A, Jouve A. Type A behavior pattern in a screened female population. Adv Cardiol 1982; 29: 96–107.

[22] Haynes SG, Feinleib M, Levine S, Scotch N, Kannel WB. The relationship of psychosocial factors to CHD in the Framingham Study II. Prevalence of CHD. Am J Epidemiol 1978; 107: 384–402.

[23] Jenkins CD, Zyzanski SJ, Rosenman RH. Progress toward validation of a computer-scored test for the type A coronary-prone behavior pattern. Psychosom Med 1971; 33: 193–202.

[24] Matthews KA, Krantz DS, Dembroski TM, Macdougall JM. Unique and common variance in structured interview and Jenkins Activity Survey measures of the type A behavior pattern. J Pers Soc Psychol 1982; 42: 303–13.

[25] Schucker B, Jacobs DR Jr. Assessment of behavioral risk for coronary risk for coronary disease by voice characteristics. Psychosom Med 1977; 39: 219–28.

[26] Haynes SG, Levine S, Scotch N, Feinleib M, Kannel WB. The relationship of psychosocial factors to CHD in the Framingham study I. Methods and risk factors. Am J Epidemiol 1978; 107: 362–83.

[27] Haynes SG, Feinleib M. Type A behavior and the incidence of CHD in the Framingham Heart Study. Adv Cardiol 1982; 29: 85–94.

[28] Kannel WB, Feinleib M. Natural history of angina pectoris in the Framingham study. Am J Cardiol 1972; 29: 154–63.

[29] Bengtsson C, Hällström T, Tibblin G. Social factors, stress experience, and personality traits in women with ischemic heart disease, compared to a population sample of women. Acta Med Scand 1973; suppl 549: 82–92.

[30] Kenigsberg D, Zyzanski SJ, Jenkins CD, Wardwell WI, Licciardello AT. The coronary-prone behavior pattern in hospitalized patients with and without CHD. Psychosom Med 1974; 36: 344–51.

[31] Blumenthal JA, Williams RB, Kong Y, Schanberg SM, Thompson LW. Type A behavior pattern and coronary atherosclerosis. Circulation 1978; 58: 634–9.

[32] Frank KA, Heller SS, Kornfeld DS, Sporn AA, Weiss MB. Type A behavior and coronary angiographic findings. J Am Med Assoc 1978; 240: 761–3.

[33] Silver L, Jenkins CD, Ryan TJ, Melidossian C. Sex differences in the psychological correlates of cardiovascular diagnosis and coronary angiographic findings. J Psychosom Res 1980; 24: 327–34.

[34] Williams RB Jr, Haney TL, Lee KL, Kong YH, Whalen RE. Type A behavior, hostility, and coronary atherosclerosis. Psychosom Med 1980; 42: 539–49.

[35] Bass C, Wade C. Type A behaviour: Not specifically pathogenic. Lancet 1982; 2: 1147–9.

[36]Abbott AR. Presence of coronary artery disease in Type A women. Ann Arbor: University of Pittsburgh, 1983. (Thesis)

[37]Pearson TA. Risk factors for arteriographically defined coronary artery disease. Ann Arbor: Johns Hopkins University, 1983. (Thesis)

[38]Haynes SG, LaCroix L, White A, Tyroler HA. The Type A-atherosclerosis controversy. Am J Epidemiol 1984: 120.

[39]Chesney MA, Black GW, Chadwick JH, Rosenman RH. Psychological correlates of the type A behavior pattern. J Behav Med 1981; 4: 217–29.

[40]Manuck SB, Craft S, Gold KJ. Coronary-prone behavior pattern and cardiovascular response. Psychophysiology 1978; 15: 403–11.

[41]Lane JD, White AD, Williams RB Jr. Cardiovascular effects of mental arithmetic in Type A and Type B females. Psychophysiology 1984; 21: 39–46.

[42]Frankenhaeuser M, Lundberg U, Forsman L. Dissociation between sympathetic-adrenal and pituitary-adrenal responses to an achievement situation characterized by high controllability: Comparison between type A and type B males and females. Biol Psychol 1980; 10: 79–91.

[43]Frankenhaeuser M. The role of peripheral catecholamines in adaption to understimulation and overstimulation. In: Serban G, ed Psychopathology of human adaptation. New York, London: Plenum Press, 1976: 173–92.

[44]Haynes SG, Feinleib M. Women, work and coronary heart disease: prospective findings from the Framingham Heart Study. Am J Public Health 1980; 70: 133–41.

[45]Haynes SG, Eaker ED. The effect of employment, family, and job stress on coronary heart disease patterns in women. In: Gold EB, ed. The changing risk of disease in women: an epidemiologic approach. Lexington, Mass: Collamore Press, 1984: 37–48.

[46]Karasek R, Baker D, Marxer F, Ahlbom A, Theorell T. Job decision latitude, job demands, and cardiovascular disease: a prospective study of Swedish men. Am J Public Health 1981; 71: 694–705.

[47]Kobasa SC, Maddi SR, Zola MA. Type A and hardiness. J Behav Med 1983; 6: 41–51.

[48]Smith TW, Houston BK, Zurawski RM. The Framingham Type A Scale and anxiety, irrational beliefs, and self-control. J Human Stress 1983; 9: 32–7.

[49]Gilbert DG, Reynolds JH. Type A personality: correlations with personality variables and nonverbal emotional expressions during interpersonal competition. Pers Individ Diff 1984; 5: 27–34.

[50]Caplan RD, Cobb S, French JRP, Van Hausen R, Dinneau SR. Job demands and worker health, main effects, and occupation differences. U.S. Department of Health, Education, and Welfare, DHHS, CDC, NIOSH, April 1975.

[51]House JS, McMichael AJ, Wells JA, Kaplan BH, Landerman LR. Occupational stress and health among factory workers. J Health Soc Behav 1979; 20: 139–60.

[52]Chesney MA, Sevelius G, Black GW, Ward MM, Swan GE, Rosenman RH. Work environment, type A behavior, and coronary heart disease risk factors. J Occup Med 1981; 23: 551–5.

[53]Frankenhaeuser M. Psychobiological aspects of life stress. In: Levine S, Ursin H, eds. Coping and health. New York, London: Plenum Press, 1981: 203–23.

[54]Karasek RA, Schwartz J, Theorell T, Pieper C, Russell S, Michela J. Job characteristics, occupation and coronary heart disease. New York: Columbia University, Department of Industrial Engineering and Operations Research, 1982.

[55]LaCroix A, Haynes SG. Occupational exposure to high demand/low control work and CHD incidence in the Framingham cohort. Am J Epidemiol 1984; 120.

[56]Haw MA. women, work and stress: a review and agenda for the future. J Health Soc Behav 1982; 23: 132–44.

Discussion on chapter 7

Bengtsson
Are there differences between men and women concerning the prevalence of behaviour A?

Haynes
The preliminary indications are that the type A behaviour pattern is only slightly more predominant in men than women—about 55–75% and 45–50% respectively.

de Faire
If you try to modify type A behaviour, are there any differences in women and men?

Haynes
My first answer would be to question the premise that we must attempt to change individual behaviour. I do not think we should attempt behaviour modification of the basic type A behaviour of men and women. There has been only one study in the United States attempting to change type A behaviour in men who have already had a myocardial infarction, to see if such a change affects the recurrence of coronary heart disease. In this study by Dr Friedman they have been able to change the speed and impatience component of type A behaviour in men. They were not able to change the overall type A behaviour pattern.

Wilhelmsson
In women, angina pectoris but not myocardial infarction was associated with behaviour pattern A. Similar findings regarding psychological stress were made among men in Göteborg.

Haynes
There is a hot reactor theory that suggests that type As are overreactors in general. If you are an overreactor, and have some pain in your chest, you might overreact to it or recognise it sooner. If you are a type A, then you may be more likely to see a physician because the pain prevents you from doing your work. We found in an angiography study at Duke University that among men who have angiography 80% are type A; among women who come in for angiography, 70% are type A.

We have examined 467 women in the Duke angiography study. Figure 7.6 shows their characteristics. They were aged 35–74 between 1978 and 1981. The structured interview measure of type A behaviour pattern was significantly related to 50% or more occlusion in one or more arteries in women but only among women aged 35–44. In the women aged 45–64, type A behaviour was not associated with the degree of coronary artery occlusion. So, in answer to the question about whether type A behaviour is related to disease in the presence of angina, the answer is yes for younger women but no for older women.

Weir
You mentioned that the women who were widowed or divorced or separated were more likely to develop coronary artery disease and that women who suppressed

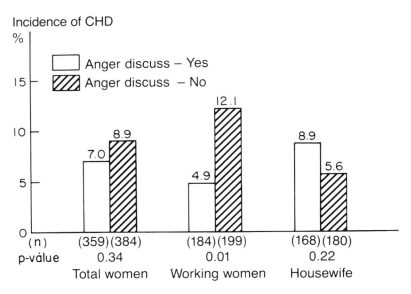

Fig. 7.6 Frequency of women with > 50% occlusion in one or more arteries. Structured interview.

anger and hostility were also at risk. If you gave these women the opportunity to talk about anger and hostility is there any evidence that this would diminish their risk?

Haynes
We classified women according to whether or not they discussed their anger. If women did discuss their anger, particularly working women, the incidence rates of coronary heart disease were significantly lower than for women who did not discuss their anger (Fig. 7.7). In fact, among men, not letting anger out was an important risk factor for coronary heart disease in white-collar men. Among women, in Framingham, not discussing anger was a more important risk factor for working women than for housewives.

Weir
Was there any relationship with those who were widowed, separated or divorced?

Haynes
We have not actually looked at the association of suppressed anger to the incidence of coronary heart disease among divorced, separated or widowed women.

Shapiro
Am I correct in thinking that you did the personality score measurement at the ninth examination, whereas the patients were classified as to coronary health status at entry much earlier in the study. Is it not conceivable that someone who starts developing, for example, vague chest pain, or tingling in the fingers long before diagnosis might perceive of himself as having his symptoms because he is inclined to drive himself fast or to eat his food fast? His symptoms and self-perception may influence the formal diagnosis of angina pectoris.

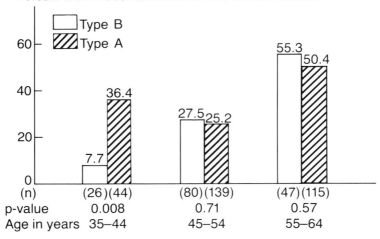

Fig. 7.7 Anger discuss among women.

Haynes

There are two theories regarding the type A behaviour of men. One suggests that the type A man denies symptoms until he becomes afflicted with disease. The other theory is that as soon as the type A man feels symptoms he attempts to seek medical care. In Framingham we eliminated persons from the prospective analysis who had any coronary disease at baseline and followed the disease-free group for 10 years. We have eliminated persons with frank disease from the population under study.

Shapiro

But, as we know, the early symptoms of coronary artery disease would not be classified as angina in any standardised procedure such as that used by the Framingham project.

Haynes

Epidemiologists have some scepticism about self-reported symptoms of that type. They are generally classified as psychosomatic problems that really have not been shown to be oetiologically related to coronary disease.

Shapiro

I am suggesting that it could be that the type A association with coronary heart disease may be spurious, that it may be accounted for by early atypical symptoms of coronary artery disease.

Haynes

I do not know of any evidence indicating this, one way or the other. I would also argue that if this is the case, we can use type A behaviour, at least in the clinical setting, to identify high-risk individuals who are more likely to progress to coronary disease. I would like to see some biological explanation for type A association. A finding like your suggestion would require further investigation.

Currently, type A investigators are trying to refine type A behaviour in an attempt to answer the question of what behaviour explains the type A-coronary heart disease association-suppressed anger, lack of control. Secondly, we are interested in the biological mechanism.

Robertson
In what proportion of people did you find difficulty in giving a classification of A or B?

Haynes
Well, in terms of the Framingham type A scale and all the other self-reported measures like those used in Jenkin's activity scale, they agree only about 60–70% of the time with structured interview. What is the valid standard if the structured interview is not relevant for the classification of type A behaviour in women?

Robertson
That was not quite my question. Did you have to discard a proportion because of difficulty in classification?

Haynes
We examined the entire Framingham scale for each sex/age group. Those in the upper 50% of scores for each age/sex group were classified as type A in the diagrams. Those in the lower 50% of scores were classified as type Bs. We have also examined the data with the type A scale as a continuous measure. As such, type A behaviour is also significantly associated with coronary disease in the logistic aggression analysis. The preference for analysis is to use the type A scale as a continuous variable, which assumes that there is a range of various degrees of type A behaviour.

Robertson
Well, I agree with that. Would it not therefore be more revealing if you could plot the incidence of complications in relation to that continuous variable?

Haynes
The sample size prohibited us from presenting the data in a continuous fashion. At one point, we analysed the data into thirds, the upper third, middle and lower third of type A scores. This was about as far as we could divide the denominators in order to have an adequate number of cases for the incidence rates. There was a dose-response relationship.

Wynn
Can you just confirm that in terms of type A there is a greater risk in the higher scores?

Haynes
Yes, in my paper for this conference I have reviewed all the prevalence studies and case control studies as well as the angiography studies, and there is overwhelming

evidence from at least 13 published papers that high scores on type A measures are associated with the prevalence of coronary heart disease, and with the degree of coronary artery disease as measured in angiographic studies.

Rifkind
Firstly, would you like to comment on the MRFIT data which did not apparently identify type A as a risk factor, and, secondly, how would you deal with the suggestion that, within the Framingham study, you have not really related type A behaviour to a reliable endpoint? Angina is obviously a soft endpoint. It has predictive value but it is undoubtedly weaker. Might you be uncovering non-ischaemic heart disease subjects who are reporting symptoms mistaken as angina related to their behaviour?

Haynes
The MRFIT findings released at the American Heart Association Council on Epidemiology meetings in 1983 showed that there was no association in men between type A behaviour and subsequent mortality. This was a group of high-risk men, as based on the standard coronary risk factors. I cannot explain the negative findings. There is also another negative study from the AMIS, Aspirin Myocardial Infarction studies. Among high-risk men, no association was found between type A behaviour with subsequent mortality in that trial.

The type A investigators are re-examining the MRFIT data, and are rescoring a sample of the interviews with the hypothesis that hostility was related to subsequent mortality but not overall type A behaviour. One thought is that the structured interviews given in MRFIT were not administered in the same manner as they were administered in the 1950s, when Friedman and Rosenman developed the type A behaviour interview. The early interviews were more hostile in nature. Over time, the epidemiologists may have asked for a less hostile interview, since study subjects might not return if a hostile interview was given. Thus, if the style of interviewing changes, and hostility was the basis of type A behaviour in men, we would not all find an association. If we reclassify the MRFIT individuals according to how much hostile behaviour they showed during the interview, we may see different results. The other possibility is that type A behaviour is not a risk factor among high-risk men, or among white-collar men.

Rifkind
You have not answered the question on angina.

Haynes
Regarding angina pectoris as endpoint among women under the age of 65 years who developed angina, 75% had abnormal or borderline ECG findings between examinations 8 and 12; among all comparably aged women in the Framingham cohort, an average abnormality rate of 17% at any one exam is experienced. The abnormalities included non-specific T- or S-T-wave changes, intraventricular block, left ventricular hypertrophy, atrioventricular conduction disturbances, atrial fibrillation or flutter, or less of QRS potentials. These findings indicate that the clinical diagnosis of angina in women is accompanied by ECG findings of coronary disease.

Bengtsson

Have you found any difference between premenopausal and postmenopausal women?

Haynes

The Framingham women were of postmenopausal age, 45–77 years.

8. Association between menopause and risk factors for ischaemic heart disease

C. Bengtsson, L. Lapidus and O. Lindquist

It has long been a matter of controversy whether or not early menopause is a risk factor for ischaemic heart disease (IHD). When the literature was reviewed some years ago[1] most papers reported such a connection, but other studies did not. The results from more recent studies are still being disputed. Thus Gordon et al[2] reported from the Framingham Study an increased risk and Rosenberg et al[3] also reported an increased risk, but Jullien et al[4] and Blanc et al[5] did not. From another series Rosenberg et al[6] even reported a decreased risk for IHD in women with early menopause.

Any such relationship might be caused by the menopause per se or it might be secondary to factors which influence the menopause.[7] Depending on the connection between the menopause and such risk factors, these factors might either increase or decrease the risk of IHD.

This paper will present results from a longitudinal population study of women in Göteborg, Sweden, which has been going on since 1968, with respect to the menopause in relation to IHD and to risk factors for IHD.

STUDY POPULATION

A population sample of 1462 women in all was studied in Göteborg, Sweden in 1968–69. Because of the sampling process and the high participation rate (over 90%) the participants were known to be representative of all women of the same ages in the community. At the time of the study they were aged 38, 46, 50, 54, or 60. They were restudied 6 and 12 years later—in 1974–75 and 1980–81. Further details about the studies have been given previously.[8–10]

All women in Göteborg who had myocardial infarction (MI) during the years 1968–70 and who were of similar age to the participants in the population study were included in a separate study.[1]

METHODS

In each of the three examinations the women were interviewed about menstrual status. From postmenopausal women information was obtained concerning the time of their last menstruation. Women who had had no menstruation for a period of 6 months or longer were defined as postmenopausal. The interview also included questions about gynaecological surgery.

The diagnosis of MI was based on chest pain, transaminases and ECG findings.[1] Angina pectoris was defined according to Rose.[11] Body weight was measured to the nearest 0.1 kg, the subjects wearing only briefs. Blood pressure was measured using a mercury sphygmomanometer to the nearest 2 mm Hg. Phase 5 of the diastolic blood pressure was registered. Laboratory examinations included serum cholesterol and serum triglycerides. Details about these laboratory examinations have been given previously.[12] Information about smoking habits was obtained by interview.

Statistical methods

The significance of differences between mean values was estimated with Student's t-test. The hypothesis of no difference in frequences between groups was tested with the chi^2-test. Differences were considered statistically significant for values of $p < 0.05$. Analysis of correlation between variables in the initial study and endpoints when confounding variables were taken into account were performed by means of Pitman's permutation test.[13]

RESULTS

Menopausal age in relation to IHD

Case control study
Ten of 46 women (22%) had their menopause at the age of 45 or earlier in the group of women who had MI during the years 1968–70, compared with 67 of 578 (12%) in a reference group consisting of participants of similar ages in the population study in 1968–69. The difference was statistically significant ($p < 0.05$). Five of 28 women (18%) with angina pectoris had their menopause at the age of 45 or earlier, which was not significantly different from the reference group. Menopause at the age of 50 or earlier was reported by 28 of 37 women with MI (76%, $p < 0.001$) and in 14 of 22 women with angina pectoris (64%, $p < 0.05$) compared with 280 of 578 women (48%) in the reference group. Further details have been reported in a previous monograph.[1]

Longitudinal study
The women in the population sample were also followed in a prospective study which consisted of the 12 year period between 1968–69 and 1980–81. When studied by means of a non-parametric permutation test[13] there was no significant correlation between premature menopause (here defined as menopause at the age of 45 or earlier) and MI, whether or not surgical menopause was included. There was, however, a significant correlation between premature spontaneous menopause and angina pectoris according to our preliminary results.

Menopausal age in relation to risk factors for IHD
The cross-sectional results presented here about smoking habits, arterial blood

pressure, body weight, serum cholesterol and serum triglycerides are confined to women in the population sample who were 50 years of age at the time of the study in 1968–69. The longitudinal data are confined to women who were 46 years old in 1968–69 and thus aged 52 at the time of the second study in 1974–75.

Smoking habits

80 of 161 menopausal 50 year-old women (50%) were smokers compared with 43 of 168 premenopausal women (26%). The difference was highly significant (p < 0.001). The postmenopausal smokers had on average smoked as long as, or longer, than the smokers who still menstruated. The high number of smokers among postmenopausal women could not be explained by these women starting to smoke in connection with the menopause. Non-smoking women were, on average, heavier than smoking women. Previous studies indicate that an increased amount of adipose tissue might delay the menopausal age.[14] It seemed, however, that smoking per se was the main factor for the early menopause. Detailed results have been presented in a previous paper.[15]

Cross-sectional data on blood pressure, body weight and serum lipids

Table 8.1 shows means of blood pressure, body weight and serum lipids in premenopausal and postmenopausal 50 year-old women. Women who had their menopause because of surgery are not included. There were statistically significant differences for all these variables except for diastolic blood pressure. Serum cholesterol and serum triglycerides were higher in postmenopausal than in premenopausal women, while the opposite was found for systolic blood pressure and body weight.

Table 8.1 Serum cholesterol, serum triglycerides, arterial blood pressure and body weight in menstruating premenopausal (n=164) and postmenopausal (n=162) 50 year-old women.

| | Premenopausal | | Postmenopausal | | Statistical |
	Mean	SD	Mean	SD	significance
Serum cholesterol (mmol/l)	6.90	0.96	7.42	1.19	p < 0.001
Serum triglycerides (mmol/l)	1.14	0.49	1.34	0.64	p < 0.001
Systolic blood pressure (mm Hg)	140	22	135	21	p < 0.05
Diastolic blood pressure (mm Hg)	86	10	86	11	NS
Body weight (kg)	681.	11.2	64.4	10.3	p < 0.001

NS=no statistical significance

Table 8.2 shows serum cholesterol and serum triglyceride levels in postmenopausal 50 year-old women in relation to postmenopausal time. There was a tendency for increased serum lipids with increasing postmenopausal time, which means that women who had their menopause early had higher serum lipids than postmenopausal women with late menopause. In this respect there was also a similar trend, but in the opposite direction, for blood pressure and body weight.

In a similar way remaining premenopausal time could be related to the serum lipids in 50 year-old premenopausal women. This was possible because information

Table 8.2 Serum cholesterol (mmol/l), serum triglycerides (mmol/l), arterial blood pressure (mm Hg) and body weight (kg) in women aged 50 (studied in 1968–69) in relation to postmenopausal time.

Time after menopause (months)	Serum cholesterol			Serum triglycerides		Systolic BP		Diastolic BP		Body weight	
	n	Mean	SD	Mean	SD	Mean	SD	Mean	SD	Mean	SD
1–5	38	7.07	0.89	1.32	0.58	140	24	85	10	68.3	14.2
6–11	28	7.12	1.25	1.30	0.81	137	16	86	7	65.5	10.3
12–23	42	7.36	1.39	1.33	0.70	134	22	85	11	65.6	12.6
24–35	31	7.37	1.15	1.33	0.65	140	22	89	12	65.1	9.8
36–59	33	7.53	0.94	1.29	0.41	134	27	84	13	62.0	8.2
≥ 60	28	7.74	1.11	1.47	0.60	129	13	84	8	63.7	9.4

Table 8.3 Serum cholesterol (mmol/l), serum triglycerides (mmol/l), arterial blood pressure (mm Hg) and body weight (kg) in women aged 50 (studied in 1968–69) in relation to remaining premenopausal time.

Time before menopause (months)	Serum cholesterol			Serum triglycerides		Systolic BP		Diastolic BP		Body weight	
	n	Mean	SD	Mean	SD	Mean	SD	Mean	SD	Mean	SD
0–5	17	6.81	0.85	0.89	0.20	134	19	84	10	68.4	15.1
6–11	10	7.05	1.07	1.05	0.21	138	23	87	11	65.7	7.4
12–23	33	6.71	0.83	1.07	0.36	139	22	87	12	66.5	10.5
24–35	32	6.96	0.99	1.22	0.75	136	26	83	11	65.4	9.3
36–59	32	6.95	0.86	1.25	0.56	146	18	88	9	71.9	13.3
≥ 60	7	7.21	0.97	1.25	0.23	143	18	84	11	64.4	7.3

about menopausal age was obtained in 1974–75 from women who stopped menstruating during the 6 year period between 1968–69 and 1974–75. There were no clearcut trends when these variables recorded in 1968–69 were related to remaining premenopausal time (Table 8.3)

Longitudinal data on blood pressure, body weight and serum lipids
One group of women who were premenopausal in 1968–69 had still not stopped menstruating in 1974–75 (group A in Fig. 8.1). Women in another group were premenopausal in 1968–69 but stopped menstruating during the period between the two studies (group B in the figure). A third group consisted of women who were postmenopausal on both occasions (group C). Of the women who were 46 years of age at the time of the initial study and thus 52 when restudied in 1974–75, 53 were to be included in group A, 193 in group B and 32 in group C. Changes in body weight, serum cholesterol and serum triglycerides in the three groups are presented in Figure 8.2. There was an increase both in serum cholesterol and serum triglycerides in the group of women in whom menstruation stopped during the period. These changes were statistically significant. There was also a statistically significant

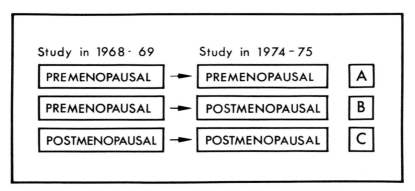

Fig. 8.1 Grouping (groups A, B and C) according to menopausal state at the time of the studies in 1968–69 and 1974–75.

increase in body weight in this group during the period, while there was a (statistically non-significant) decrease in body weight in women who were already postmenopausal at the time of the first examination.

A significant rise in blood pressure with age was observed in women with unchanged menstrual status (groups A and C) but not in those women who had become postmenopausal between the two examinations (group B).

It is therefore obvious that there is a relationship between the menopause and factors such as blood pressure, body weight and serum lipids as observed by us when studied both cross-sectionally and longitudinally. Further details from the studies of these relationships have been presented previously.[7,12,16]

DISCUSSION

Any definite statement about whether there is a relationship between menopausal

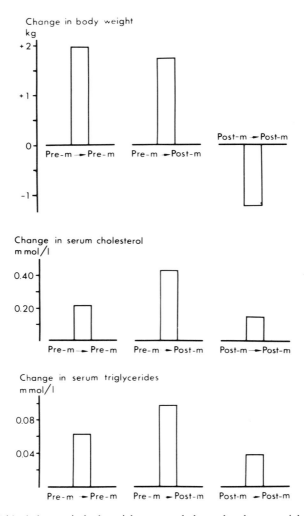

Fig. 8.2 Intraindividual changes in body weight, serum cholesterol and serum triglycerides in relation to change (or no change) in menopausal status.

age and IHD cannot yet be given. The results from different studies are still contradictory. Even so, there is no doubt that there is an association between the menopause and different risk factors for IHD such as blood pressure, serum cholesterol, serum triglycerides and smoking habits. It is also a matter for discussion whether increased body weight is to be considered as a risk factor for IHD. In a study of men in Göteborg an increased waist/hip quotient has been found to be a risk factor for MI,[17] and similar as yet unpublished results have been obtained in our prospective study of women. Willett et al[18] found an association between relative weight and menopausal age but after adjustment for cigarette consumption the relationship was weak. There are reasons why we have included body weight in this paper. It seems obvious that the effect on menopausal age is secondary to smoking habits with a precocious menopause in smoking women compared with non-smokers.[18-22] On the other hand, it is reasonable to believe that the changes in blood pressure, body weight and serum lipids are secondary to changed menopausal state. The most pronounced differences in connection with change in menopausal state were found for serum cholesterol and serum triglycerides. These variables moved in a direction which is considered to be disadvantageous for the subject. The influence on blood pressure and body weight seemed to be in the opposite direction and should therefore be advantageous for the subject. Different relationships have been summarised in Figure 8.3. With respect to all different associations, often with probable effects in both directions, it is easy to understand why the relationship between menopausal age and IHD may be complex and that results from such studies in the future might also be contradictory.

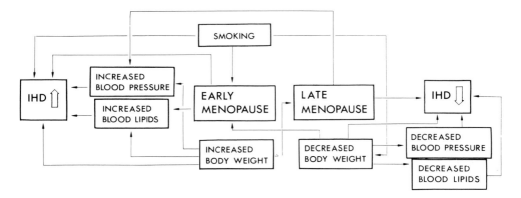

Fig. 8.3 Possible interrelationships between menopausal age, ischaemic heart disease (IHD), body weight, smoking habits, serum lipids and arterial blood pressure. From Lindquist and Bengtsson.[15]

SUMMARY

There are still contradictory opinions about whether or not there is an association between menopausal age and ischaemic heart disease. In a cross-sectional study we have found an increased number of women with early menopause in a group of women who had myocardial infarction (MI), but this finding could not be confirmed when we carried out a prospective study. There is no doubt, however, that there are associations between menstrual status and risk factors for ischaemic heart disease (IHD). Hence, smoking gives rise to earlier menopause, while the menopause will give rise to increased serum cholesterol and serum triglyceride levels, but influence arterial blood pressure and body weight in the opposite way. The relation between the menopause and risk factors for IHD is complex, which may be one explanation for the contradictory results when associating menopausal age with IHD.

ACKNOWLEDGMENT

The analyses and presentation of data were supported by grants from the Swedish Medical Research Council 27X-4578.

REFERENCES

[1]Bengtsson C. Ischaemic heart disease in women. A study based on a randomized population sample of women and women with myocardial infarction in Göteborg, Sweden. Acta Med Scand 1973; suppl 549.

[2]Gordon T, Kannel WB, Hjortland MC, McNamara PM. Menopause and coronary heart disease. The Framingham study. Ann Intern Med 1978; 89: 157–61.

[3]Rosenberg L, Hennekens CH, Rosner B, Belanger C, Rothman KJ, Speizer FE. Early menopause and the risk of myocardial infarction. Am J Obstet Gynecol 1981; 139: 47–51.

[4]Jullien G, Gichtenaere JC, Gerard R. Coronary insufficiency in the female: possible effect of menopause. Nouv Presse Med 1977; 6: 1125–8.

[5]Blanc JJ, Boschat J, Morin JF, Clavier J, Penther P. Menopause and myocardial infarction. Am J Obstet Gynecol 1977; 127: 353–5.

[6]Rosenberg L, Miller DR, Kaufman DW et al. Myocardial infarction in women under 50 years of age. JAMA 1983; 250: 2801–6.

[7]Lindquist O. Influence of the menopause on ischaemic heart disease and its risk factors and on bone mineral content. Acta Obstet Gynecol Scand 1982; suppl 110.

[8]Bengtsson C, Blohmé G, Hallberg L et al. The study of women in Gothenburg 1968–1969— a population study. General design, purpose and sampling results. Acta Med Scand 1973; 193: 311–8.

[9]Bengtsson C, Hallberg L, Hällström T et al. The population study of women in Göteborg 1974–1975—the second phase of a longitudinal study. General design, purpose and sampling results. Scand J Soc Med 1978; 6: 49–54.

[10]Sigurdsson JA. High blood pressure in women. A cross-sectional and a longitudinal follow-up study. Acta Med Scand 1983; suppl 659.

[11]Rose GA. The diagnosis of ischaemic heart pain and intermittent claudication in field surveys. Bull WHO 1962; 27: 645–58.

[12]Lindquist O, Bengtsson C. Serum lipids, arterial blood pressure and body weight in relation to the menopause: results from a population study of women in Göteborg, Sweden. Scand J Clin Lab Invest 1980; 40: 629–36.

[13]Bradley JV. Distribution-free statistical tests. Englewood Cliffs, NJ: Prentice-Hall, 1968.

[14]Daniell HW. Osteoporosis of the slender smokers. Vertebral compression fractures and loss of metacarpal cortex in relation to postmenopausal cigarette smoking and lack of obesity. Arch Intern Med 1976; 136: 298–304.

[15]Lindquist O, Bengtsson C. Menopausal age in relation to smoking. Acta Med Scand 1979; 205: 73–7.

[16]Lindquist O. Intraindividual changes of blood pressure, serum lipids, and body weight in relation to menstrual status: results from a prospective population study of women in Göteborg, Sweden. Prev Med 1982; 11: 162–72.

[17]Larsson B, Svärdsudd K, Welin L, Wilhelmsen L, Björntorp P, Tibblin G. Abdominal adipose tissue distribution, obesity, and risk of cardiovascular disease and death: 13 year follow-up of participants in the study of men born in 1913. Br Med J 1984; 288: 1401–4.

[18]Willett W, Stampfer MJ, Bain C et al. Cigarette smoking, relative weight, and menopause. Am J Epidemiol 1983; 117: 651–8.

[19]Jick H, Porter J, Morrison AS. Relation between smoking and age of natural menopause. Lancet 1977; 1: 1354–5.

[20]Adena MA, Gallagher HG, Cigarette smoking and the age at menopause. Ann Hum Biol 1982; 9: 121–30.

[21]Andersen FS, Transbol I, Christiansen C. Is cigarette smoking a promotor of the menopause? Acta Med Scand 1982; 212: 137–9.

[22]Goulding A. Smoking, the menopause and biochemical parameters of bone loss and bone turnover. NZ Med J 1982; 95: 218–20.

Discussion on Chapter 8

Oliver

The question whether the effects of the menopause are due to the menopause or due to a change in risk factors might be studied by looking at the pattern of coronary heart disease when there was a very early menopause. I refer to some of our early work looking at the effect of the menopause before the age of 35. In women who developed secondary amenorrhoea in their 20s or who had bilateral oophorectomy, there was a greater-than-expected increase in coronary heart disease over the next 20 year-period and we were not able to find any change in the pattern of risk factors.

Sternby

I suppose that when there is a very early menopause it is common to introduce oestrogen treatment. What happens if you treat women for 10–15 years with oestrogen?

Oliver

I am referring to two studies which were done before it was common to introduce oestrogen. I have no idea what the effect would be of giving oestrogen.

Slack

Dr Bengtsson, what is your definition of the menopause? You seem to use a specific moment in time.

Bengtsson

We asked the women when they had their last menstruation. We repeated the same questions 6 years later. It appeared that if a woman had had no menstruation for half a year, the chance of her menstruating again was small. Postmenopausal women were defined as having had no menstruation during the last 6 months.

Rosenberg

It seems to me that the evidence linking the risk of myocardial infarction to menopause is very weak. A curve of the log of the rate of coronary death in women according to age does not have a difference in the rate of change through the menopausal years. In addition, you mentioned a number of articles relating menopause to myocardial infarction. I think that most of these studies are flawed in one way or another. I myself have participated in two studies of menopause and myocardial infarction. One showed that menopause was harmful, the other showed it might actually be protective. I am rather agnostic.

Haynes

The menopause was related to angina. What does the diagnosis of angina pectoris mean in women?

Bengtsson

That is a difficult question. We don't know what it means, but angina pectoris in women seems not to be the same as angina pectoris in men. However, the survival rate in women with myocardial infarction and men with myocardial infarction is about the same. When we compare the survival rate of women and men with angina pectoris there is a substantial difference. Women will survive much longer than men. I think that many of the women, although fulfilling the requirements of the Rose questionnaire, do not have ischaemic heart disease.

Haynes
If this conference could answer that one question, we would be making a major contribution to the medical community which is confounded by the issue.

Vedin
In trying to go further in describing female angina pectoris we will soon run into problems. The meaning of a so-called positive exercise ECG is totally different among women than among men. The relationship between any given coronary angiographic anatomy and the response in terms of exercise ECG is totally unpredictable.

Bengtsson
About 10% of the women had a history of angina pectoris and changes in the ECG indicating ischaemic heart disease when performing an exercise test.

Haynes
In the United States, 50% of women who go to angiography have no occlusion or stenosis. Either we are doing too many procedures on women or women have some type of pain that has nothing to do with atherosclerosis of the major arteries. Perhaps the pain has something to do with another anatomical abnormality.

9. Adverse metabolic effects of oral contraceptives

V. Wynn

The subject of this paper is those metabolic changes which may have aetiological significance in the cardiovascular problems produced by oral contraceptives in young women. The clinical condition of most concern is myocardial infarction (MI) which, together with cerebrovascular disease, has become the single most obtrusive severe complication of oral contraceptive use. In a conference in 1977 in Edinburgh I gave a paper[1] with a similar title to the present paper, and then reviewed what was known about the metabolic effects of oral contraceptives in relation to the problem of interest, namely, coronary heart disease in young women. The main emphasis was on the changes in carbohydrate and lipid metabolism produced by oral contraceptives and the conclusion I reached was: 'It is therefore important for doctors to be cautious in the prescription of oral contraceptives and to try to identify on clinical grounds alone those women for whom this sort of medication could be potentially dangerous and at the same time to prescribe contraceptive formulations which produce the minimum of metabolic effect, avoiding especially oral contraceptives containing high doses of oestrogen.'

One can see from this that the recommendation was to avoid pills containing high oestrogen content, and later I will show a review of the biochemical findings as they appeared at that time which gave weight to this opinion. But it is of interest that my conclusion in the present paper will be that it is important to avoid the use of oral contraceptives which contain progestins stronger than are necessary to give good contraceptive protection and menstrual cycle control. In other words, the metabolic emphasis has gone in a complete circle, focusing attention away from the oestrogen and concentrating on the progestin. The reasons for this are twofold: first, along with the realisation of the thrombotic potential induced by the biochemical changes which were under oestrogen control—especially changes in blood clotting factors— oral contraceptives have progressively been introduced with lower and lower oestrogen content so that pills containing 100 μg oestrogen, which were common in the USA until recently. Second, with the progressive lowering of the oestrogen dosage, the manufacturers have increased the strength of the progestin in order to give greater contraceptive protection and to improve menstrual cycle control. In 1981 a symposium was held in London, the title of which was: 'Progestogens and the cardiovascular system'.[2] Several contributors discussed the epidemiological evidence that related high progestin dosage to unwanted cardiovascular complications in the use of oral contraceptives—especially hypertension, MI, and cerebrovascular disease. Another important consideration was the knowledge that the strong progestins used in the low oestrogen dose oral contraceptives was lowering the level of the serum high-density lipoproteins (HDL), and especially the protective HDL-2 fraction,[3] and that they were also causing increased insulin resistance and hyperinsulinaemia. Finally, data from my laboratory[4] showed that there was a progressive deterioration in glucose tolerance over a period of 3 years in a group of women using one of the new low-dose combined oral contraceptives, namely a pill containing 30 μg oestrogen and 150 μg levonorgestrel. This effect drew attention to yet another undesirable feature of using over-strong progestogens in oral contraceptives.

TYPES OF PROGESTIN USED IN ORAL CONTRACEPTIVE FORMULATIONS

Three main classes of progestins are currently used in combined oral contraceptives, namely the oestranes, the gonanes, and the pregnanes.

Oestrane progestins are all related to norethisterone and include norethisterone acetate, lynoestranol, norethynodrel, and ethynodiol diacetate. Norethisterone is the active substance and the other compounds mentioned must be converted by metabolic transformation into norethisterone before they become active.

The second class of progestins are the gonanes, the main representative of which is norgestrel which is similar to norethisterone in structure except that its methyl substituent is replaced by an ethyl group. Norgestrel is much more potent weight for weight than norethisterone and, by some criteria—for example, its effect on serum HDL levels—it is about ten times as strong. It is totally synthesisable and is therefore a compound of great interest to the pharmaceutical industry. The active component of norgestrel is the dextro-isomer, levonorgestrel. This is not always made clear in the metabolic literature, but the reader needs to know that norgestrel consists of an equal mixture of d- and l-isomers, the l-form being inactive. When doses of norgestrel are referred to throughout this presentation it means the dose of levonorgestrel.

A recent modification of norgestrel has been the introduction of the compound desogestrel which is similar to norgestrel except for a methylene substituent on the 11-carbon of the steroid ring. This modification is said to render the drug less androgenic while retaining its powerful progestogenic activity. Metabolic information available so far is insufficient to draw a firm conclusion about this aspect.

The third class of progestins, namely the pregnanes, are derivatives of 17-hydroxyprogesterone and they are: chlormadinone, megestrol, and cyproterone acetate. The first two progestins mentioned are no longer used in oral contraceptives because of untoward pharmacological effects in beagle dogs, but cyproterone acetate is becoming popular because it is a fairly strong antiandrogen and oral contraceptives containing it are said to be useful in the management of hirsutism and acne in women requiring contraceptive protection.

COMBINED ORAL CONTRACEPTIVE FORMULATIONS

The past 25 years or so of combined oral contraceptive medication have seen a continuing development of formulations including various amounts of oestrogen* (from 150 μg to 20 μg ethinyloestradiol) and varying combinations and doses of the three classes of progestins described above. In addition to the fixed combinations of steroids there have been attempts to introduce regimens in which the amount of oestrogen and/or progestin varies with varying phases of the cycle. These phasic types of oral contraceptives are achieving greater popularity in certain countries, including the UK, but the amount of clinical and metabolic information available about them is still too limited to assess their advantages and disadvantages. In what follows, therefore, the description of the metabolic changes produced by oral contraceptives will refer exclusively to the use of fixed-dose formulations.

We have studied seven main groups of combined oral contraceptives, namely:

1. high oestrogen (75 μg to 150 μg ethinyloestradiol) combined with an oestrane progestin
2. medium oestrogen (50 μg ethinyloestradiol) combined with a pregnane progestin
3. medium oestrogen combined with an oestrane progestin
4. medium oestrogen combined with 250 μg levonorgestrel
5. low oestrogen (30 μg) combined with 250 μg levonorgesrel
6. low oestrogen (30 μg ethinyloestradiol) combined with 150 μg levonorgestrel
7. low oestrogen (20 μg ethinyloestradiol) combined with 1 mg norethisterone acetate

GLUCOSE TOLERANCE, SERUM INSULIN, AND BLOOD PYRUVATE LEVELS IN ORAL CONTRACEPTIVE USERS

Figure 9.1 shows the changes in glucose tolerance with corresponding serum insulin and blood pyruvate levels in a group of women tested before and during the administration of a variety of combined oral contraceptives. When these studies were carried out we were not familiar with the concept that various oral contraceptives may have different effects on carbohydrate metabolism, so the changes observed were the mean result observed in this group of women.

They show impairment of glucose tolerance in the users with raised serum insulin and blood pyruvate levels. These changes are identical with those observed in patients taking small doses of glucocorticoids and for this reason we referred to these effects as 'steroid diabetes'. Using the area under the glucose tolerance curve but above the fasting value (the incremental area) as a single index of the rate of glucose dissimilation we showed that the greatest deterioration in glucose tolerance was found with a high oestrogen pill but the greatest increase in insulin secretion was found with a pill containing levonorgestrel (Fig. 9.2). This study showed that

*Two oestrogens are used in the oral contraceptive formulations—mestranol and ethinyloestradiol. The former is converted quantitatively to the latter compound before it is active. The metabolic effects of these two compounds are identical.[2]

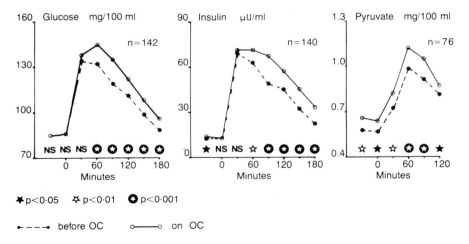

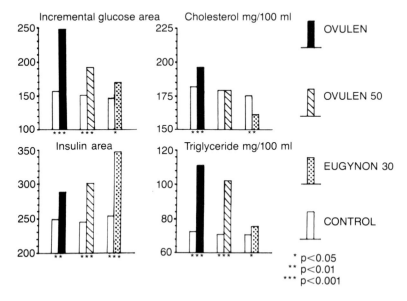

Fig. 9.1 Oral glucose tolerance, plasma insulin, and blood pyruvate levels in women before and on various oral contraceptives (OC). Conversion to SI units: glucose 1 mg/100 ml=0.0555 mmol/l.

there were significant differences between the various formulations of combined oral contraceptives in respect of carbohydrate metabolism. Figure 9.2 also shows that the high-oestrogen pill was associated with significantly raised cholesterol and triglyceride levels, whereas the norgestrel-containing pill was associated with a significantly lowered serum cholesterol and only moderately raised serum triglyceride. It was the combination of the various effects shown in Figure 9.2 which led us to make the recommendation previously referred to that high-oestrogen pills should

Fig. 9.2 Glucose, insulin and lipid parameters in women taking three groups of combined oral contraceptives. Conversion to SI units: cholesterol 1 mg/100 ml=0.0259 mmol/l; triglyceride 1 mg/100 ml=0.0112 mmol/l.

106

not be used, and preference should be given to pills containing 30 μg oestrogen which, at the time these studies were done, was invariably associated with a gonane progestin. We did not realise at the time that the low serum cholesterol was due to a lowering of the HDL cholesterol, an effect which can hardly be described as beneficial. Neither did we place much emphasis on the increased insulin secretion found with the norgestrel-containing pill. Subsequently our interpretation of these data suggested that, on metabolic grounds alone, of the three pills reported here the one to be preferred would be the medium oestrogen combined with the oestrane progestin.

COMPARISON OF EFFECTS ON CARBOHYDRATE METABOLISM OF SIX GROUPS OF COMBINED ORAL CONTRACEPTIVES

Figure 9.3 summarises our metabolic findings in subjects taking six groups of the combined pills referred to above. The numbers of subjects in each group are shown. It can be seen that most of the pills significantly lower fasting plasma glucose and impair glucose tolerance, the greatest effect being with the high-oestrogen pill. Insulin secretion is increased but this is most obvious with the three combined pills containing levonorgestrel. The ratio of insulin area to glucose area (an index of insulin resistance) shows that the levonorgestrel-containing pills cause greater insulin resistance than the other combined pills. Figure 9.3 also gives the effects of the various combined oral contraceptives on serum cholesterol and serum triglyceride and shows that the norgestrel-containing pills cause greater insulin resistance than the other combined pills. Figure 9.3 also gives the effects of the various combined oral contraceptives on serum cholesterol and serum triglyceride and shows that the norgestrel-containing pills lowered the serum cholesterol and had the least effect on fasting serum triglyceride.

LONGITUDINAL STUDIES OF EFFECTS OF COMBINED ORAL CONTRACEPTIVES ON CARBOHYDRATE METABOLISM

A low-dose levonorgestrel-containing pill

The studies just reported were carried out in a cross-sectional manner—that is to say, women were tested while taking various combined oral contraceptives and their results were compared with a control group of non-users. This is the simplest way to carry out metabolic studies but it is not necessarily the most sensitive test of the metabolic effect of various compounds. We decided, therefore, to study the effects on carbohydrate metabolism in a group of women acting as their own controls. They had glucose tolerance with insulin measurements done before taking the pill and then at 3 months, 1 year, 2 years, and 3 years of use in order to produce a series. [2-5] Figure 9.4 shows the effects on glucose tolerance (glucose area and incremental glucose area) in a large group of women taking a pill containing 30 μg ethinyloestradiol and 150 μg levonorgestrel. It can be seen that there is a progressive deterioration in glucose tolerance with time—the trend being significant ($p < 0.01$). The numbers on the horizontal axis refer to the number of cases tested at each time interval and the data displayed refer only to the data of the individuals as they

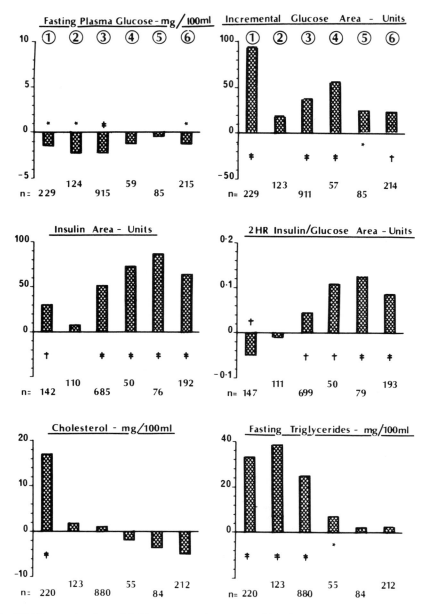

Fig. 9.3 Glucose, insulin and lipid parameters in women taking six groups of combined oral contraceptives.

completed each duration of the study. There has been a progressive attenuation of the number of subjects as is to be expected in studies of this sort which consists of young women of high mobility. Nevertheless, the internal consistency of the results is remarkable.

Figure 9.5 shows the corresponding insulin secretion in this group of subjects:

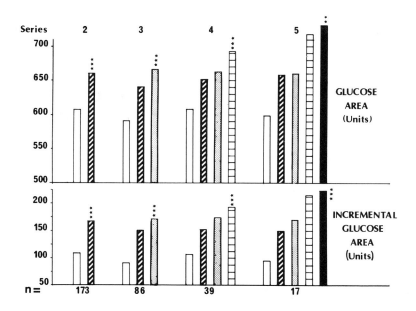

Fig. 9.4 Glucose tolerance parameters in women taking 30 μg ethinyloestradiol and 150 μg levonorgestrel.

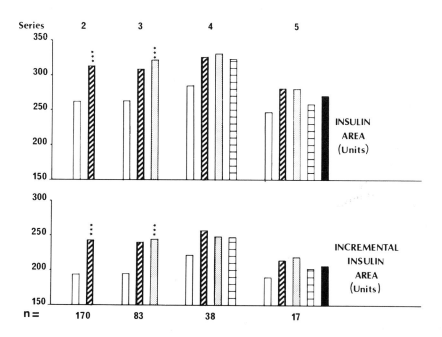

Fig. 9.5 Insulin parameters during glucose tolerance test in women taking 30 μg ethinyloestradiol and 150 μg levonorgestrel.

there is an initial increase in insulin secretion at 3 months but thereafter there is no significant change. Figure 9.6 shows the change in the ratio of incremental insulin area to incremental glucose over the series. It can be seen that there is a progressive decrease in this ratio (p<0.01) which implies that the initial pancreatic response is unable to keep pace with the increasing insulin resistance so that there is progressive glucose tolerance deterioration without a corresponding increase in insulin secretion. This is the metabolic change which one finds in many cases of subclinical diabetes. These data are reported in greater detail elsewhere.[4]

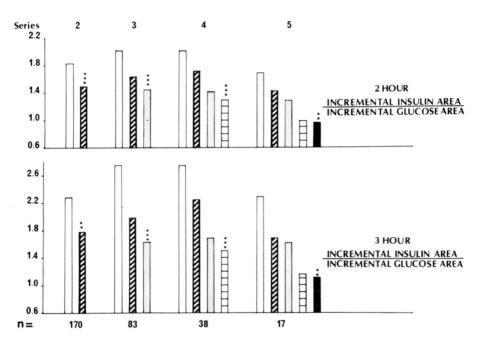

Fig. 9.6 Incremental insulin area/incremental glucose area ratio in the same group of women as in Figs. 9.4 and 9.5.

A low-dose norethisterone-containing pill

In contrast to these findings we have studied another group of women in an identical manner using a combined pill which contains 20 μg oestrogen and 1 mg norethisterone acetate. Figure 9.7 shows a moderate deterioration in glucose tolerance at 3 months, but thereafter no progressive change over a period of 3 years. The women also show a moderate increase in insulin secretion which remains constant throughout the 3 year period of observation (Fig. 9.8). The insulin/glucose ratio falls at 3 months and thereafter remains unchanged (Fig. 9.9). When the two types of pill studied here are compared using percentage changes from baseline values, it can be clearly seen that the largest percentage change in glucose tolerance and decrease in insulin/glucose ratio occurs with the norgestrel-containing pill compared with the pill containing norethisterone (Fig. 9.10).

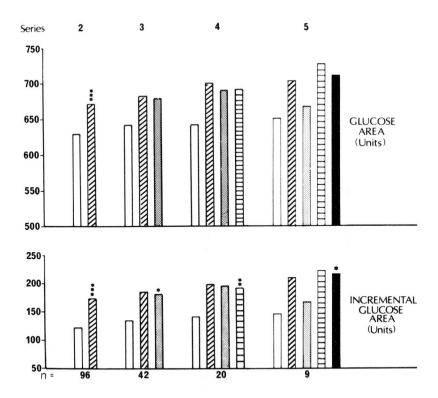

Fig. 9.7 Glucose tolerance parameters in women taking 20 μg ethinyloestradiol and 1 mg norethisterone acetate.

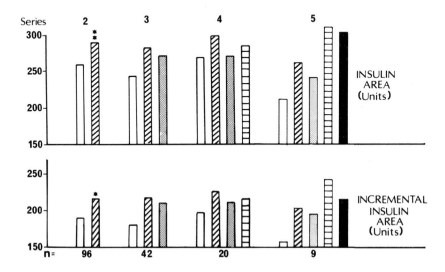

Fig. 9.8 Insulin parameters during glucose tolerance test in women taking 20 μg ethinyloestradiol and 1 mg norethisterone acetate.

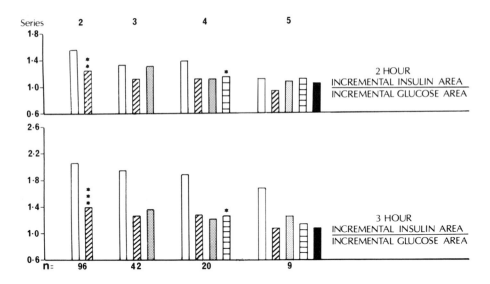

Fig. 9.9 Incremental insulin area/incremental glucose area ratio in the same group of women as in Figs. 9.7 and 9.8.

I conclude from this that even 150 µg levonorgestrel with µg ethinyloestradiol is too strongly progestogenic for continuous use in a combined pill and that over a period of 3 years it will produce progressive deterioration in glucose tolerance with inappropriately low insulin secretion. Judged by these metabolic effects this pill is not ideal for prolonged use in young women. In comparison, the combined pill containing 20 µg ethinyloestradiol and 1 mg norethisterone acetate had significantly less effect on carbohydrate metabolism.

Since insulin resistance is one of the best-documented metabolic effects of progesterone itself and is a property of many androgens and related compounds, such as the progestins used in oral contraceptives,[5] and since the clinical consequences of prolonged insulin resistance are unknown but may be related to premature atherosclerosis,[6,7] I conclude that we should use oral contraceptive formulations which cause the least insulin resistance. In this respect the norgestrel formulations studied here are less suitable than the norethisterone-containing pills that we have investigated.

EFFECTS OF ORAL CONTRACEPTIVES ON SERUM LIPIDS

Table 9.1 shows the effect of four combined oral contraceptives on serum cholesterol, triglyceride and HDL cholesterol levels compared with control subjects. The pills studied contained 30 µg ethinyloestradiol combined with 250 µg or 150 µg levonorgestrel, 50 µg ethinyloestradiol combined with 1 mg norethisterone acetate, and 20 µg ethinyloestradiol combined with 1 mg norethisterone acetate. 410 women who were not using the pill acted as controls. The subjects were well matched for age and percentage ideal body weight. They had been taking oral contraceptives for a

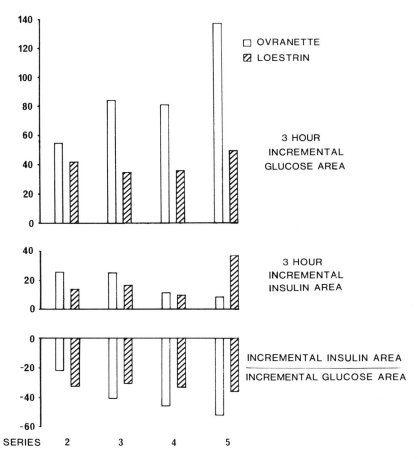

% DIFFERENCE BETWEEN PRE AND SERIES VALUES

Fig. 9.10 Comparison of percentage changes in glucose and insulin parameters between two different combined oral contraceptives, namely 30 μg ethinyloestradiol and 150 μg levonorgestrel (Ovranette), and 20 μg ethinyloestradiol and 1 mg norethisterone acetate (Loestrin).

substantial period varying from mean durations of 10–80 months. It can be seen that serum cholesterol is significantly reduced by the pills containing levonorgestrel. Serum triglyceride is increased most by the pills containing norethisterone acetate. HDL cholesterol is significantly reduced by pills containing levonorgestrel but not by the pills containing norethisterone acetate. This is especially noticeable in the Loestrin group (20 μg ethinyloestradiol, 1 mg norethisterone acetate). The difference in HDL cholesterol in this group compared with the 250 μg levonorgestrel group is 11.1 mg (25%). This difference occurs despite the fact that Loestrin contains only 20 μg ethinyloestradiol compared with 30 μg in the 250 μg levonorgestrel pill. As is well known, androgens (and androgenic progestins) lower HDL. These data suggest that levonorgestrel is a strong progestin compared with norethisterone.

Table 9.1 Serum lipids in control and combined oral contraceptive users.

	Control	EO 30 µg levoNG 250 µg	EO 30 µg levoNG 150 µg	EO 50 µg NEA 1 mg	EO 20 µg NEA 1 mg
No of cases	410	114	259	45	99
Age (years)	28.1	27.8	27.3	33.0	27.4
% ideal body weight	100.9	103.1	99.2	99.8	97.2
Duration (months)		44.7	37.5	80.6	20.5
Cholesterol (mg/100·ml)	174.9	165.0*	167.2*	183.3	179.4
Triglyceride (mg/100·ml)	62.5	63.1	69.8**	94.8**	80.1**
HDL cholesterol (mg/100·ml)	57.1	48.1**	53.0**	57.8	59.2

EO=ethinyloestradiol
levoNG=levonorgestrel
NEA=norethisterone acetate
*p < 0.01, ** p < 0.001

Table 9.2 HDL subfractions in control and combined oral contraceptive users.

	Control	EO 30 µg levoNG 250 µg	EO 30 µg levoNG 150 µg	EO 50 µg NEA 1 mg	EO 20 µg NEA 1 mg
No of cases	279	111	180	40	97
HDL$_2$ cholesterol (mg/100·ml)	24.6	19.9**	18.8**	26.5	26.4
HDL$_3$ cholesterol (mg/100·ml)	33.1	28.4**	34.6	31.4	32.6
HDL$_2$/HDL$_3$	0.83	0.83	0.60**	1.06	1.06
HDL$_2$/LDL	0.20	0.18*	0.17**	1.06	0.23

EO=ethinyloestradiol
levoNG=levonorgestrel
NEA=norethisterone acetate
LDL=low-density lipoprotein cholesterol
* p < 0.05, **p<0.001

Table 9.2 shows the effect of the four combined pills under test on HDL_2 and HDL_3 levels and on the ratio of HDL_2 to low-density lipoproteins (LDL). The pills containing levonorgestrel lower HDL_2, unlike the norethisterone acetate-containing pills, which have no effect. HDL_3 is also lowered by the pill containing 250 μg levonorgestrel. The HDL_2/LDL ratio is significantly reduced by the two pills containing levonorgestrel. This ratio is considered to be an atherogenic risk indicator when it is studied in patients not receiving medication that affects lipid levels. Although a drug-induced change in HDL and HDL_2 levels cannot be evaluated with certainty because evidence is incomplete, nevertheless it is wisest to regard these changes produced by steroid drugs as being potentially harmful until proved otherwise.

Table 9.3 Serum lipids and HDL subfractions in control and progestogen-only oral contraceptive users.

	Control	NG 75 μg	NEA 350 μg
No of cases	68	26	26
Age (years)	27.4	33.2	32.6
% ideal body weight	105.8	97.6	100.1
Duration (months)		54.2	42.5
Cholesterol (mg/100 ml/100 ml)	179.1	175.2	175.0
Triglyceride (mg/100 ml)	64.6	66.1	66.7
HDL cholesterol (mg/100 ml)	59.8	51.8*	58.1
HDL_2 cholesterol (mg/100 ml)	25.2	20.0	24.6
		(p=0.08)	
HDL_3 cholesterol (mg/100 ml)	34.6	31.8	33.5

NG=norgestrel (equivalent to 37.5 μg levonorgestrel)
NEA=norethisterone acetate
*$p < 0.05$

Table 9.3 shows the effect on serum lipids, including HDL and HDL subfractions of progestogen-only oral contraceptives. It can be seen that HDL cholesterol is significantly reduced by norgestrel (37.5 μg levonorgestrel) but not by norethisterone acetate in a tenfold higher dose. This suggests that, as far as the effect on serum lipids is concerned, levonorgestrel is about ten times more potent than norethisterone.

CONCLUSION

These studies on the effect of various combined oral contraceptives on carbohydrate and lipid metabolism show that various effects are found according to the dose of oestrogen and the type and dose of progestin. The combination of drugs which would produce the least untoward effect on the parameters studied here is a pill containing 30–35 μg oestrogen with 1 mg norethisterone acetate. It may be possible to improve further on the metabolic profile while retaining good contraceptive efficacy and cycle control by using phasic formulations of these drugs, but only further research will determine whether or not this is the case.

REFERENCES

[1] Wynn V. Metabolic effects of oral contraceptives in relation to coronary heart disease in young women. In: Oliver MF, ed. Coronary heart disease in young women. Edinburgh, London, New York: Churchill Livingstone, 1978: 129–37.

[2] Symposium: Progestogens and the cardiovascular system. London 17–18 July 1981. Am J Obstet Gynecol 1982; 142: 717–816.

[3] Wynn V, Niththyananthan R. The effect of progestins in combined oral contraceptives on serum lipids with special reference to high-density lipoproteins. Am J Obstet Gynecol 1982; 142: 766–72.

[4] Wynn V. Effect of duration of low-dose oral contraceptive administration on carbohydrate metabolism. Am J Obstet Gynecol 1982; 142: 736–46.

[5] Effect of progesterone and progestins on carbohydrate metabolism. In: Bardin CW, Milgröm E, Mauvais-Jarvis P, eds. Progesterone and progestins. New York: Raven Press, 1983: 395–410.

[6] Stout R.W. The relationship of abnormal circulating insulin levels to atherosclerosis. Atherosclerosis 1977; 27: 1–13.

[7] Orchard TJ, Becker DJ, Kuller LH, Wagener DK, LaPorte RE, Drash AL. Age and sex variations in glucose tolerance and insulin responses: parallels with cardiovascular risk. J Chronic Dis 1982; 35: 123–32.

116

Discussion on chapter 9.

Bengtsson

Dr Weir and Dr Wynn—have you any comments on the discrepant effects of oestrogens and progestins on blood pressure and other factors?

Wynn

The oestrogens obviously have an effect on blood pressure; the progestins also have an effect on blood pressure but it is different from that of oestrogen. Furthermore, you have got the changes in clotting factors probably due to changes in the prostaglandins caused by oestrogen. There are also changes in lipids and carbohydrate metabolism produced by progestins and then all these factors may interreact within each other.

Weir

Have you any information about metabolic changes with desogestrel combinations and triphasic combinations?

Wynn

The information is very scanty. There are just not enough studies of the metabolic effects. There has been no time yet to assess the clinical safety of the new products. Studies of several thousand patients for a number of years are needed.

Oliver

With preparations where the oestrogen content has been steady, namely 30 μg, and the progesterone content has decreased, has there been any change in any of the thrombosis parameters?

Wynn

This is one of those strangely difficult questions. This study cannot be done in the United States where they have large numbers of subjects but either because many of the newer preparations are not available or because they are not popular with the physicians the answer to that question will not be obtained in the United States for quite a long time. In England we only have the general practitioner study. This study stopped recruiting subjects soon after the introduction of the low-oestrogen products so it is unlikely to produce reliable data because of insufficient numbers. Another British study (Oxford-FPA study) is still continuing. Professor Vessey who runs it has the impression that cardiovascular side effects may be being reduced by lowering the progestin and the oestrogen.

Oliver

Because, as one uncovers the oestrogen effect, one might expect a greater thrombotic effect.

Wynn

Are we talking about venous thrombosis or arterial thrombosis?

Oliver
I am talking about the haemostatic variables that are measured in vitro.

Wynn
Yes, I think the haemostatic variables will go up as you uncover the oestrogen effect. And that introduces a balance into the equation and only time will tell. When you are dealing with five or six variables you realise how difficult it is to get them all right simultaneously. Then you have got the variable of the woman—what the woman wants is a safe contraceptive and, more than anything, she wants regular cycles. You cannot convince a woman to take a pill that gives her nearly 100% contraceptive protection and irregular cycles; she won't have it.

10. Continued effects of oral contraceptives after cessation of treatment

S. Shapiro

In 1981 we published the results of a case-control study suggesting that the protracted use of oral contraceptives may continue to confer an increased risk of myocardial infarction (MI) when their use is ended.[1] The risk following protracted use appeared to persist for as long as 5–9 years.

Actually, in preliminary analyses we had found that the overall rate ratio for discontinued oral contraceptive use (last use more than 1 month previously) was 1.2. The result was not statistically significant. We found, as had others,[1,2] that current oral contraceptive use was associated with a threefold to fourfold increase in the risk. We assumed that the underlying mechanism was an increased tendency to thrombosis that subsided quite promptly when use ended, and we did not explore the data for possible duration effects associated with discontinued use.

We were stimulated to examine the duration effects of discontinued oral contraceptive use only after Dr Bruce Stadel of the National Institutes of Health and Professor Victor Wynn of St Mary's Hospital, London, suggested that we do so. They, in turn, had been stimulated by the mounting body of evidence[2] that oral contraceptive use changes lipid patterns, and other risk factors, in ways that might be expected to increase the risk of MI—especially if those changes are sustained over many years.

In this presentation I will refer to the salient results concerning discontinued oral contraceptive use and consider some of the issues that they raise.

PATIENTS AND METHODS

The methods have been described.[1] For completeness they are given here almost verbatim, but omitting most references to current oral contraceptive use.

A case-control study was conducted. Data were collected between 1 July 1976 and 30 June 1979.

To identify cases of MI the coronary care units of 155 hospitals in Greater Boston, Long Island and the coastal area north of New York City, and in the Delaware Valley were telephoned, usually at weekly intervals. Whenever a woman below the age of 50 years was admitted, the physician was contacted and asked whether the patient had a definite MI. When the diagnosis was affirmed, a nurse-interviewer questioned the patient during convalescence in the hospital or, if she had already been discharged, at home. The nurses also interviewed five or more potential control patients in the same hospitals.

At the interview, menopausal status was determined, and detailed medical histories (particularly about risk indicators for MI) were obtained, as were comprehensive histories of drug use. The women were asked whether they had ever taken medication for contraception, regulation of periods, menstrual problems, breast conditions, endometriosis, sexual difficulties, or for any gynaecological reason. The time and duration of use were recorded. Whenever the patient knew the brand name of the oral contraceptive, it was recorded. Photographs of packets of pills were provided to aid recall when necessary.

The interview was refused by the patient or physician in 6% of both the cases and the potential control subjects.

Case series

There were 613 women below the age of 50 years who did not have a history of MI and who were diagnosed by the attending physicians as having a definite infarction. We reviewed the clinical records of 559 (91%), 54 of whom were excluded from further consideration either because they did not meet the World Health Organization criteria for the diagnosis[3] (31), or because of prior coronary bypass surgery, cardiac valve prosthesis, rheumatic heart disease, occurrence of infarction after admission, or sickle-cell crisis preceding the infarction (23).

When the clinical record was not available (54 patients), the physician's diagnosis was accepted. Among the 559 remaining women, only three were below 25 years of age and they were also excluded, leaving a final series of 556 cases 25–49 years of age who sustained a first episode of MI. The median age was 44 years.

Control series

Women were considered eligible as potential control subjects if they were 25–49 years of age, if they did not have a history of MI, and if the reason for admission was judged to be unrelated to the prior use of oral contraceptives. Subjects admitted for certain chronic debilitating conditions or their complications (rheumatoid arthritis, cancer, and so on) were not considered eligible. There were 3841 women. From among them, control subjects were selected at random so that the ratio of controls to cases was 4:1 within 5 year age groups, with the exception of 45–49,years: for 290 cases in this age group, only 972 control subjects were available (ratio, 3.4:1). The final control series thus consisted of 2036 women. The median age was 44 years.

The primary condition for which the controls were admitted was of sudden and recent onset (acute) among 639 women (31%) (Table 10.1), of whom 391 were admitted for trauma and 248 for infections. The remaining 1397 controls (69%) were admitted for less acute conditions. Orthopaedic diagnoses accounted for 618 patients, of whom 511 had disc disease or low back pain. A wide variety of conditions accounted for the remaining 779 admissions.

Past oral contraceptive use of any duration (last use more than 1 month before admission) was reported by 57% of controls between the ages of 25 and 39 years, and by 42% and 26% in the age groups 40–44 and 45–49 years. For past use that lasted 5 or more years, the corresponding percentages were 12, 10 and 6.

Table 10.1 Past oral contraceptive (OC) use in controls.

		No of patients	Past OC use*		Past OC use for 5 or more years*	
			No	(%)	No	(%)
Age (years)	25–29	44	25	(57)	5	(11)
	30–34	120	70	(58)	14	(12)
	35–39	272	152	(56)	35	(13)
	40–44	628	262	(42)	65	(10)
	45–49	972	253	(26)	56	(6)
Primary diagnosis						
1. Acute	Trauma	391	158	(40)	36	(9)
	Infection	248	75	(30)	17	(7)
2. Non-acute	Orthopaedic	618	244	(39)	60	(10)
	Other	779	285	(37)	62	(8)
Total		2036	762	(37)	175	(9)

* Last use at least 1 month before admission

Rates of any past use and past use for 5 or more years were similar among all the diagnostic categories in the control series. This uniformity persisted on standardisation for age.

There were 41 cases (7%) and 51 controls (3%) who had used oral contraceptives within a month of admission (current use); they are omitted from further consideration in this report.

Analysis

Two analytic approaches were used as appropriate. In the first, age alone was controlled; the data were stratified by half-decade of age, and rate ratios were estimated with the Mantel-Haenszel method;[4] 95% confidence limits were computed with Miettinen's test-based method.[5]

The second approach was based on multiple logistic regression.[6] Indicator terms for the following potential confounding factors were included jointly in the equations: location of the hospital, age, ethnic group, cigarette smoking, hypertension, lipid abnormality, preeclamptic toxaemia, diabetes mellitus, angina pectoris, ponderal index (weight/height[2]), and menopausal status. Indicator terms were also used for oral contraceptive use, including the date of the last use and the total duration of use. The relation of MI to the duration of use was also evaluated in terms of ordinal variables scaled to test for trend.

RESULTS

The frequencies of past oral contraceptive use among cases and controls are given in Table 10.2. For past oral contraceptive use overall, the rate ratio estimate was 1.2, with 95% confidence limits of 0.9 and 1.4 (multivariate estimate, 1.1; 95% confidence limits, 0.9 and 1.4). On confining the analysis to those who did not have predisposing conditions (Table 10.3), the rate ratio estimate for past use was 1.3 (0.9 and 1.7).

The duration of past oral contraceptive use is considered in Table 10.4. The information was sparse for subjects under 40 years of age. For subjects who were at

Table 10.2 Frequenies of past* oral contraceptive (OC) use in cases of myocardial infarction (MI) and controls.

Age (years)		Total no of subjects	Past OC use* No exposed	Rate ratio	None** No of subjects
25–34	MI	41	14	0.7	11
	Controls	164	95		49
35–44	MI	225	103	1.1	108
	Controls	900	414		462
45–49	MI	290	89	1.3	190
	Controls	972	253		712
	Overall rate ratio estimate +			1.2	
	(95% confidence limits)†			(0.9–1.4)	

* Last use at least 1 month before admission
** Reference category
+ Adjusted for half-decade of age
† 95% confidence limits

Table 10.3 Frequencies of past* oral contraceptive (OC) use in cases of myocardial infarction (MI) and controls without known predisposing conditions**

Age (years)		Total no of subjects	Past OC use* No exposed	Rate ratio	None** No of subjects
25–34	MI	22	6	0.7	5
	Controls	155	87		48
35–44	MI	114	56	1.2	49
	Controls	716	332		360
45–49	MI	142	50	1.6	86
	Controls	727	196		525
	Overall rate ratio estimate+			1.3	
	(95% confidence limits)			(0.9–1.7)	

* Last use at least 1 month before admission
** Excludes history of hypertension, lipid abnormality, diabetes and angina
+ Adjusted for half-decade of age and smoking status

Table 10.4 Distribution of cases of myocardial infarction (MI) and controls according to duration of past* oral contraceptive (OC) use.

Age (years)		Duration of past OC use* (years) < 5	5–9	≥ 10	Unknown	Never used OCs
25–39	MI	35	9	3	3	37
	Controls	176	46	8	17	153
Rate ratio estimate**		0.8	0.8	1.5	–	(1.0)+
40–49	MI	93	32	25	6	272
	Controls	362	81	40	32	1070
Rate ratio estimate**		1.0	1.6	2.5	–	(1.0)+

* Last use at least 1 month before admission
** Adjusted for half-decade of age
+ Reference category

least 40 years of age the rate ratio increased with increasing duration of past use, and the trend[7] was statistically significant ($\chi^2_1 = 12.1$, p<0.01; multivariate test for trend (p<0.01). The rate ratio for 10 or more years use was 2.5 (p<0.05). With the analysis in this age category confined to those without predisposing conditions (Table 10.5), the trend[7] was again evident and statistically significant ($\chi^2_1 = 7.2$, $p<0.01$). The rate ratio for 10 or more years' use was 3.0 ($p<0.05$).

Table 10.5 Distribution of cases of myocardial infarction (MI) and controls according to duration of past* oral contraceptive (OC) use. Subjects without known predisposing conditions.** Age 40–49 years.

| | Duration of past OC use* (years) | | | | |
	< 5	5–9	≥ 10	Unknown	Never used OCs
MI	51	16	18	3	122
Controls	281	65	31	24	802
Rate ratio estimate ***	1.1	1.5	3.0	–	(1.0) ±

* Last use at least 1 month before admission
** Excludes history of hypertension, lipid abnormality, diabetes and angina
*** Adjusted for half-decade of age and smoking status
+ Reference category

Table 10.6 Relation of myocardial infarction (MI) to past* oral contraceptive (OC) use for 5 or more years according to time elapsed since last use. Age 40–49 years.

Time elapsed since last OC use (years)	MI	Controls	Rate ratio estimate †	(95% confidence limits)
Never used OCs	272	1070	(1.0) +	
5	24	53	1.8	(1.1–3.0)
5–9	26	43	2.5	(1.5–4.1)
≥ 10	5	17	1.2	(0.4–3.2)
Unknown	2	8	–	–
Total	57	121	1.9	(1.4–2.7)

* Last use at least 1 month before admission
† Adjusted for half-decade of age
+ Reference category

Table 10.7 Relation of myocardial infarction (MI) to past* oral contraceptive (OC) use for 5 or more years according to smoking status. Age 40–49 years.

Smoking status**	Group	Duration of OC use ≥ 5 years	Never used OCs	Rate ratio estimate
Never smoked	MI	8	44	2.5
	Controls	28	350	
Ex-smoker***	MI	4	19	2.9
	Controls	14	145	
1–24 cigarettes/day	MI	17	97	1.5
	Controls	45	376	
≥ 25 cigarettes/day	MI	28	112	1.4
	Controls	32	183	

* Last use at least 1 month before admission
** Smoking status unknown in 18 controls
*** Last smoked 1 or more years before admission

The effect of the time interval after discontinuing long-term use (use that lasted at least 5 years) among women 40–49 years of age is considered in Table 10.6. The overall rate ratio estimate was 1.9, and there was no evidence of a consistent trend according to the time elapsed. However, numbers were sparse for the time interval of 10 or more years after discontinuation.

Rate ratios for the past long-term use of oral contraceptives according to cigarette smoking are given in Table 10.7. The rate ratio was highest among non-smokers (2.5 to 2.9; p<0.05) and tended to decrease according to the number of cigarettes smoked. This tendency[7] was statistically significant (p<0.01).

DISCUSSION

A full consideration of the findings in terms of validity is given in the original report,[1] and will not be repeated here. I wish only to reemphasise that the information on oral contraceptive use was based on recall in a study in which a sizeable proportion of the cases (as well as the interviewers) were aware of the hypothesis. Validation studies[8,9] suggest that oral contraceptive use is remembered with acceptable accuracy as a 'yes/no' variable. But the argument can be made that the results of this study could be spurious if the cases tended systematically to overestimate (or if the controls tended to underestimate) the duration of past use. In statistical terms, however, the magnitude of a systematic bias that would reduce the rate ratio of 3.0 to 1.0, among women not known to be predisposed to MI, would have to be very large indeed. I judge it unlikely that the association would have been eliminated had the study been demonstrably free of information bias. Until a study is done in which the recording of oral contraceptive use is not dependent on recall, the question must, however, remain unresolved. That issue aside, the findings appear to be consistent with what might be expected on biological grounds.

I should like next to consider an important methodological issue concerned with the epidemiological exploration of the aetiology of common diseases, using MI as a model. This is a theme that will be developed further in Chapter 12, and one that is now becoming a major concern in epidemiological research in general.

The problem can be stated simply: when findings in any reasonably well-conducted study suggest that the risk of a disease appears to be increased several-fold by some 'exposure' (such as high cholesterol), bias of some type may be present, but the higher the rate ratio, the less likely is it that the complete absence of bias would eliminate the association. For a disease as common as MI, however, even an increase in the risk of the order of 20% or 30% is serious. Yet it is precisely when the estimated rate ratio is 1.2 to 1.3 that bias may most readily account for it. Moreover, although optimally conducted non-experimental research can sometimes, in theory at least, eliminate information bias and selection bias, there is always the residual possibility that a low rate ratio can be accounted for by uncontrolled, and possibly unknown, sources of confounding. Where small increments in risk are of the greatest public health importance their confident identification is the most insecure.

The situation, however, although difficult is not hopeless. One obvious strategy, of course, is to require rigorous study design and analysis before rate ratios of low magnitude can be taken seriously. The present findings suggest additional strategies that may be broadly divided, on the one hand, into sharpening the definition of the exposure of interest, and, on the other hand, into sharpening the definition of the outcome.

First, the definition of the exposure. The overall ratio for past oral contraceptive use, based on multivariate analysis, was 1.1, a result that could easily have been due to bias, confounding, or chance. A more relevant definition in biological terms, long-term use of 5 or more years' duration, increased the estimate to 1.9, and the result was now statistically significant. In addition, across three categories of increasing duration, the trend for the rate ratio to increase was also significant. Chance, as an explanation of the data, seems unlikely. Nevertheless, even an approximate doubling of the risk could still be due to bias.

Second, the definition of the outcome. Without specifying any exclusions, the rate ratio for 10 or more years' duration of past oral contraceptive use was 2.5, but when the analysis was confined to cases and controls not known to be predisposed to MI, and hence at a lower baseline risk of a disease with a multifactorial aetiology, it increased to 3.0.

Another convenient way to identify varying levels of baseline risk is to classify subjects according to smoking status: since it has been shown that about two-thirds of MI in women below the age of 50 years is due to cigarette smoking.[10] In this study, the risk declined significantly from a rate ratio of 2.5 to 2.9 among non-smokers down to 1.4 among heavy smokers.

Thus, restricting the analysis to exposures that are substantial and to domains of low basline risk enables the identification of rate ratio estimates high enough (of the order of 2.5 to 3.0) to reduce concerns about bias or confounding. Such concerns are obviously substantial when the overall rate ratio estimates are as low as 1.1 or 1.2, as in the present example.

Of course, women below the age of 50 years are, to begin with, at low baseline risk for MI. This is itself an advantage: the evaluation of MI in that domain can serve to identify aetiological factors that might otherwise be obscured when the disease is explored in a domain of more common occurrence, where many other competing risk factors may also be present. This topic will be considered again in relation to variables other than oral contraceptives by Dr Rosenberg. But here it is worth making the general point that in trying to decide whether a rate ratio of a low order of magnitude for a common disease represents cause and effect, it may be worth exploring domains in which the occurrence of the disease is rare: a substantially increased risk in the rare domain may serve to strengthen a causal inference for a modestly increased risk in the common domain.

Some qualifications are in order. Firstly, sharpening the definition of exposure may not always be helpful. In the present context, for example, it is known that current oral contraceptive use increases the risk of thrombosis throughout the cardiovascular system;[2] yet there is no duration effect. It would be odd, however, if the risk were to decline, rather than remain the same, with increasing duration of use. In the present study, current oral contraceptive use was associated with about the same level of risk (presumably via thrombogenic mechanisms) regardless of duration of use.[1] On the other hand, duration of past use (as against duration of current use) was relevant—suggesting that in deciding how to sharpen the definition of exposure, biological considerations may be helpful.

Secondly, findings identified within domains of low baseline risk in which a disease is uncommon (such as the occurrence of MI in young women) may not necessarily be applicable in generalizing to domains of high risk with common occurrence, since it may be that we are examining diseases that are ostensibly the same but actually different. In addition, if different risk factors modify each other's action, exploration in a rare domain may or may not prove to be helpful. It can be helpful if two factors augment each other's effects, as with the combination of cigarette smoking and current (but not past) contraceptive use (Table 10.8);[11] it can be misleading if two factors tend to neutralise each other—in this last instance, however, I am unable to give a quantitative example.

There is one further methodological consideration. The exploration in rare domains of diseases that occur commonly in other domains almost invariably necessitates a case-control approach. Moreover, within such explorations, there is a further need to subclassify the exposure, as well as the baseline risk—and, in addition, to attain adequate numbers within relevant strata. It follows that studies must be designed to be much larger than would simply be necessary to obtain an overall result that is statistically significant.

In the present study, over 600 cases of a rare disease were enrolled. Even that number was insufficient to determine whether protracted oral contraceptive use continues to confer an increased risk of MI a decade or more after use has ended. The most important public health question in the entire study remained unanswered. A relatively large increase in the incidence of a rare disease poses no serious problems, but if protracted oral contraceptive use continues to confer an increased risk of MI up to ages when the disease becomes common, a serious hazard exists.

Table 10.8 Separate and combined effects of current oral contraceptive (OC) use and cigarette smoking in relation to myocardial infarction: age-adjusted rate ratio estimates (95% confidence limits).[11]

Cigarette smoking	OC use	
	No	Yes
None	(1.0)[+]	4.5 (1.4–14.1)
1.24	3.4 (2.2–5.1)	3.7 (1.0–13.2)
> 25	7.0 (5.2–11.5)	39 (22–70)

[+]Reference category
≥

SUMMARY

The results (previously reported) of a case-control study of the risk of myocardial infarction (MI) after ending oral contraceptive use in 40–49 year-old women yielded an overall rate ratio of 1.1; over categories of oral contraceptive use that lasted less than 5 years, 5–9 years, and 10 or more years, the rate ratio estimate increased from 1.0 to 1.6 to 2.5 (p<0.01). In the absence of known predisposition (other than smoking) to MI, the corresponding estimates were 1.1, 1.5, and 3.0 (p<0.01).

For common diseases, small increments in risk may be important, but it is often difficult to ensure that such increments are not due to bias or chance. The model of MI in young women illustrates strategies that may be helpful in coping with this problem. These strategies include sharpening the definition of the exposure (based on biological considerations), and the exploration of the disease in domains of low baseline risk (such as in young non-smoking women). If a high rate ratio is uncovered in the rare domain, a causal inference for a lower rate ratio estimate in a domain of common occurrence may be strengthened.

126

ACKNOWLEDGMENT

This study was supported by a contract (N01-HD-6-2849) from the National Institute of Child Health and Human Development, a contract (223-76-3016) from the Food and Drug Administration, and a grant-in-aid from Hoffmann-La Roche, Inc.

REFERENCES

[1] Slone D, Shapiro S, Kaufman DW et al. Risk of myocardial infarction in relation to current and discontinued use of oral contraceptives. N Engl J Med 1981; 305: 420–4.

[2] Stadel BV. Oral contraceptives and cardiovascular disease. N Engl J Med 1981; 305: 612–8; 672–7.

[3] Ischaemic Heart Disease Registers. Report of the Fifth Working Group. Copenhagen: World Health Organization, 1971.

[4] Mantel N, Haenszel W. Statistical aspects of the analysis of data from retrospective studies of disease. J Natl Cancer Inst 1959; 22: 719–48.

[5] Miettinen O. Estimability and estimation in case-referent studies. Am J Epidemiol 1976; 103: 226–35.

[6] Armitage P. Statistical methods in medical research. New York: John Wiley, 1971: 319–20.

[7] Mantel N. Chi-square tests with one degree of freedom; extensions of the Mantel-Haenszel procedure. J Am Stat Assoc 1963; 58: 690–700.

[8] Glass R, Johnson B, Vessey M. Accuracy of recall of histories of oral contraceptive use. Br J Prev Soc Med 1974; 28: 273–5.

[9] Stolley PD, Tonascia JA, Sartwell P E et al. Agreement rates between oral contraceptive users and prescribers in relation to drug use histories. Am J Epidemiol 1978; 107: 226–35.

[10] Rosenberg L, Shapiro S, Kaufman DW, Slone D, Miettinen OS, Stolley PD. Cigarette smoking in relation to the risk of myocardial infarction in young women. Modifying influence of age and predisposing factors. Int J Epidemiol 1980; 9: 57–63.

[11] Shapiro S, Slone D, Rosenberg L, Kaufman DW. Oral-contraceptive use in relation to myocardial infarction. Lancet 1979; 1: 743–7.

Discussion on chapter 10

Beaumont J.-L.
Must I understand that it is protective to be a heavy smoker?

Shapiro
No, not if one thinks in terms of incidence rates rather than relative risks. If you translate relative risks into incidence rates you find that if you take a relative risk of 1.5 when a disease is common, this translates into a much higher incidence rate. When a disease is rare a relative risk of 10 may translate into a lower incidence rate. The advantage of identifying a relative risk of 10 is that you can be pretty sure that bias does not fully account for it. It may be that the true relative risk is 9 or perhaps 11. But an association of that magnitude is not likely to disappear even if bias should be completely eliminated.

Haynes
I wonder how you would answer the ethical question of whether or not this drug should be completely eliminated from the market for use by women.

Shapiro
Well, I think that people engaged in research should generally refrain from making public health recommendations. If you are engaged in research, there is the risk that you may either be too partial to your own research, or you attempt to bend backwards so far that you become unnecessarily antagonistic to your own results. Public health recommendations should be made by other qualified people who can judge the quality of the work and decide what the public health implications are. In general, as a matter of public policy I am really not disturbed by a relative risk of 20 or 50 if the outcome is rare, if the drug is not commonly used, and if the disease for which it is used is serious. In the context of oral contraceptives the increase in the risk of venous thromboembolism, myocardial infarction and stroke occurs among young women among whom the baseline risk is so low that when you multiply an incidence that is close to zero by 10 you still get zero.

The public health issue, I think, hinges ultimately on the question of whether the residual risk of myocardial infarction is real and whether it continues to increase as women become older. The other compelling public health question is whether women who took other contraceptives for a long time early in their productive lives develop an increased risk of breast cancer when they pass the age of 40 or 50. Until we know the answers to those questions I don't think we can make final public health judgments about the safety or otherwise of oral contraceptives.

Oliver
Is there another alternative to a trial? We have hundreds of thousands of women taking oral contraceptives with different formulae, with different smoking habits, with different family histories, and no country in the world has established a data bank of such a magnitude that it will record this cohort of women. It should not be impossible to establish this and to follow the cohort and subcohorts forward for 20 years. I wonder if it is not our social and moral responsibility to do so.

Shapiro

A cohort study would have to be impractically large. Consider a cohort of women aged 50 years with a repeated incidence of infarction of perhaps 0.5–1% a year. Look at the number of variables we have to worry about and the number of cases we expect. The difficulties are daunting. I think we need another case control study. Based on the analogy with infectious disease epidemiology I would speculate that the risk declines as the interval from discontinuation increases.

Rosenberg

The British studies have shown that oral contraceptive users actually do better in terms of overall mortality than controls, and there are also data to show that the pill protects against ovarian cancer and endometrial cancer. So I think it is wrong simply to focus on one condition such as myocardial infarction. The risks must be weighed against the benefits.

Shapiro

I should add that the implications of findings such as ours may not be the same for different countries. In societies where there may be a substantial risk of morbidity or death if a woman conceives, an increased risk of myocardial infarction may be acceptable. I feel unqualified to make judgments. I think that the people who live locally in the various countries have to make the judgments and the decisions. The best we can do is to provide the information.

11. Postmenopausal oestrogen use and cardiovascular mortality in women

T.L. Bush, B.M. Rifkind, M.H. Criqui, L.D. Cowan, E. Barrett-Connor, J.M. Karon, R.B. Wallace and H.A. Tyroler

The question of whether postmenopausal oestrogen use influences the risk of cardiovascular disease (CVD) in women is a major public health issue in the United States for two reasons. First, CVD is the leading cause of death in women as well as in men; nearly two-thirds of all deaths in women are attributable to CVD. Second, postmenopausal oestrogen use is common among middle-aged women in the US, with estimates of the prevalence of postmenopausal use ranging from 15% to 50%.[1,2] Given the high prevalence of postmenopausal oestrogen use and the magnitude and seriousness of CVD in women, it is imperative from both a scientific and a public health perspective that the role of postmenopausal oestrogen in the development of CVD be elucidated.

Oestrogens, in addition to their function as sex hormones, have numerous physiological effects on metabolic functions which could impact on CVD risk. For example, oestrogens have been shown to modify carbohydrate metabolism,[3] to cause coagulation system changes,[4,5] and to alter lipid/lipoprotein metabolism, particularly influencing high-density lipoprotein (HDL) and low-density (LDL) levels.[6-8] Theoretically, the changes that oestrogens induce in carbohydrate metabolism and within the coagulation system could increase the risk of CVD, because oestrogens induce abnormal glucose and insulin levels and increase serum clotting factors which may increase the risk of a thromboembolic event. Hence the induction of a more 'diabetogenic state' or a 'hypercoagulable state' could cause an increased risk of CVD among women using this drug. On the other hand, oestrogens are known to increase HDL, high levels of which are protective against CVD, and to decrease LDL, high levels of which increase the risk of CVD. Thus, these changes in lipid/lipoprotein levels could theoretically protect against the development of CVD.

STUDIES OF THERAPEUTIC AND CONTRACEPTIVE OESTROGENS

Studies of oestrogen use and CVD risk in individuals other than postmenopausal women taking replacement oestrogens are conflicting. Several reports suggest an increased risk of CVD in oestrogen users, and others suggest that oestrogens are protective for CVD. One body of scientific evidence, derived primarily from studies in men with selected diseases and in younger women using oral contraceptives, suggests that oestrogen use increases the risk of CVD.

Data from the studies in men show that oestrogens, particularly when given in relatively high doses, increase the risk of a cardiovascular event. Results from two clinical trials, the Coronary Drug Project [9,10] and the Veterans Administration's studies of diethylstilboesterol (DES) and prostatic cancer,[11,12] show an increased risk of non-fatal [9,10] and fatal [11,12] CVD events in men taking these hormones. The increased cardiovascular risk seen in these studies was attributed to an increase in thromboembolic events.

The well-established finding that oral contraceptive use increases the risk of CVD in younger women (particularly in those users who smoke) also implicates oestrogens as a risk factor[13-15] for CVD. As in men, the hypothesised pathological mechanism for the increased risk in oral contraceptive users is an increase in thromboembolic events, ostensibly due to the oestrogen content of the oral contraceptives. A recent report, however, suggests that another biological agent, the progestin portion of oral contraceptives, may be responsible for the observed increased risk in oral contraceptive users.[16]

In contrast to the above findings, evidence from other sources suggests that oestrogens may protect against CVD. The observations of lower CVD rates in women than in men and the virtual absence of CVD in premenopausal women indirectly point to a protective effect of endogenous oestrogens. In addition, results of animal studies show that chicks fed oestrogens develop fewer atherogenic lesions than non-treated animals.[17,18] Furthermore, evidence from autopsy studies show that atherogenic lesions are increased in women with premenopausal oopherectomy[19,20] and aortic lesions are decreased in men treated with oestrogens.[21]

STUDIES OF OESTROGEN REPLACEMENT IN WOMEN

Despite the fact that postmenopausal or replacement oestrogens are widely used in the United States, relatively few studies have examined the specific effect of these oestrogens on CVD risk. The results of those studies are also conflicting, with several showing a significant beneficial effect of oestrogen use,[22-25] some suggesting no effect on CVD risk, [26-29] and others which show an increased risk of CVD in women using these hormones.[30-35]

A summary of those studies which clearly show a protective effect of oestrogen use is presented in Table 11.1. Nachtigall et al,[24] in a clinical trial of inpatients in a hospital for chronic diseases, reported that women assigned oestrogens experienced one-third of the occurrence of CVD of women assigned placebo (relative risk=0.33). Other researchers, [22,23,25] using several methodologies and well-defined populations, found the risk of CVD to be significantly lower among oestrogen users than among non-users. Estimates of the risk in users varied from 0.33 to 0.57 of non-users.

In several additional studies researchers observed risks for CVD in oestrogen users to be less than the risk in non-users, but usually interpreted the results as an indication of no increased risk of CVD among users. [26-29] These studies are summarised in Table 11.2. One study which showed no effect of oestrogens[26] has

Table 11.1 Studies showing a protective effect of oestrogen in women.

Study	Design	Population	Size	Endpoint	Risk estimate	Comments
Nachtigall et al 1979[24]	double-blind trial of 10 years' duration	postmenopausal inpatients, x=55 years of age, residents in hospital for chronic diseases	83 age-condition matched pairs	fatal/non-fatal MI	RR=0.33	oestrogen and progestins used together, patients with diabetes mellitus and ASHD included
Hammond et al 1979[23]	historical cohort	patients at Duke University treated with oestrogen and followed for at least 5 years	309 non-users 301 users	incident CVD	RR=0.33*	authors claim a beneficial effect of oestrogen therapy
Burch et al 1974[22]	historical cohort	all cases of women aged 25+ in one surgical practice	737 women followed for 9899 person-years	fatal CHD	RR=0.43*	control group undefined, all had had hysterectomies
Ross et al 1981[25]	case-control	members of retirement community < 80 years of age who died between 1971-1975	133 cases 133 living controls 124 deceased controls	fatal IHD	OR=0.43*(l) OR=0.57*(D)	cases were matched to both living (L) and deceased (D) controls

MI=myocardial infarction
CVD=cardiovascular disease
CHD=coronary heart disease
IHD=ischaemic heart disease

RR=relative risk
OR=odds ration
*p<0.05, risk estimate

Table 11.2 Studies showing ambiguous effects of oestrogen use in women. Abbreviations as in Table 11.1.

Study	Design	Population	Size	Endpoint	Risk estimate	Comments
Adam et al 1981[28]	case-control	all deaths in women 50–59 years in England/Wales, Nov 1978	76 cases 151 controls	fatal MI	OR=0.65*	pilot study—author concludes no evidence of increased risk
Pfeffer et al 1978[26]	case-control	women, aged 44–100 years (2874) living in retirement community	185 cases 511 controls	fatal/non-fatal MI	OR=0.68 (Current) OR=0.86 (Ever-use)	ratios computed for 'ever' used and current use; ratios adjusted for age, diabetes, hypertension
Bain et al 1981[29]	nested case-control	married nurses aged 33–35 years who responded to questionnaire	64 cases 1390 controls	non-fatal	MIOR=0.40*(0) OR=0.70 (C) OR=0.90 (E)	authors conclude that oestrogens do not increase risk in ever (E) or current (C) users, but may decrease risk in women with bilateral oophorectomy (0)
Rosenberg et al 1976[27]	case-control	hospitalised patients aged 40–75 years enrolled in Boston Collaborative Drug Surveillance Program	336 cases 6730 controls	non-fatal	MIOR=0.47* (Crude) OR=0.97 (Adjusted)	authors claim no evidence of an association: OR was < unity in 90% of patients; OR adjusted for age, hospital, hypertension, religion, coffee consumption and other CVD risk factors; 2% of cases were users.

*p < 0.05, risk estimate significantly less than 1.00

133

Table 11.3 Studies showing increased risk of oestrogen use in women. Abbreviations as in Table 11.1.

Study	Design	Population	Size	Endpoint	Risk estimate	Comments
Rosenberg et al 1980[34]	case-control	women aged 30–49 years admitted to CCUs in 155 US hospitals	477 cases 1831 controls	non-fatal	MIOR=1.0 (recent use) OR=1.2 (past use)	low prevalence of oestrogen use in both cases and controls
Petitti et al 1979[33]	nested case-control	participants aged 18–54 years in the Walnut Creek Contraceptive Drug Study	26 cases ? controls	fatal and non-fatal	OR=1.2 MI	authors claim no increased risk for oestrogen use
Gordon et al 1978[30]	prospective	women in the Framingham cohort, 40–54 years, 24 year follow-up	18 334 person-years; 36 CHD cases, 60 angina cases	CHD angina	RR=1.6(CHD) RR=2.3* (angina)	actual data for users and non-users not reported
Wilson et al 1985[35]	prospective (?)	women in the Framingham cohort, 51–83 years, followed for 8 years	1234 participants	non-fatal CVD	50%* increased risk of morbid CVD in users	specific cardiovascular diseases are not presented
Jick et al 1978[31]	case-control	subjects 39–45 years selected from 621 hospitals in the US	17 cases 34 controls	non-fatal	MIOR=7.5*	16 of 17 cases were smokers; low study participation
Jick et al 1978[32]	case-control	subjects 39–45 years selected from 621 hospitals in the US	19 cases 39 controls	non-fatal	MIOR=9.3*	large loss of cases and controls due to lack of participation

* $p < 0.05$, risk estimate significantly greater than 1.00

134

since been replicated with a more comprehensive definition of oestrogen use; this latter study now reports a significant protective effect of menopausal oestrogens.[25] In two of the reports which suggest no effect of oestrogen there is actually a reduced risk of CVD among oestrogen users. [27,28] Each of these studies used a case-control design.

Published reports that show an increased risk of CVD in women using replacement oestrogens are summarised in Table 11.3. In two of these studies [33,34] the risk in oestrogen users is slightly higher than the risk in non-users (odds ratio=1.2). The authors of both studies interpret these findings as evidence against an increased risk of CVD among oestrogen users.

Four other reports [30-32,35] from two other study populations show a significantly increased risk of CVD in women using oestrogens. An early report from the Framingham study[30] showed a relative risk of 2.3 for angina pectoris and a relative risk of 1.6 for other forms of coronary heart disease among women classified as users. A more recent study[35] found a 50% increase in CVD morbidity among women classified as users compared with non-users.

The highest risks of CVD reported for oestrogen users were found by Jick et al. [31,32] In two separate reports from the same population, they found the risk for oestrogen users to be 7.5[31] and 9.3[32] times that in non-users. A high proportion of smokers among cases (94%) and a large loss of study participants were significant problems in these case-control analyses.

Given the confusing and unresolved nature of the association of oestrogen use and CVD in women, and the potential public health impact of these drugs, we examined the association of postmenopausal oestrogen use and subsequent CVD mortality in a cohort of women who participated in the Lipid Research Clinics (LRC) Program.

METHODS

All women included in this study were participants in the LRC Prevalence Study conducted in 10 North American clinics between 1972 and 1976.[36] One of the primary purposes of the LRC Prevalence Study was to determine the association of lipid and lipoprotein patterns with coronary heart disease and other cardiovascular diseases.

A total of 26 899 white women participated in the initial LRC screening—visit 1. A 15% random sample of all visit 1 participants, plus all women with raised lipid levels or taking Lipid-lowering medications were invited to a second screening—visit 2. Over 84% of those women invited to visit 2 participated. Of the 5926 white women who were screened at visit 2, 127 or 2% were taking lipid-lowering medication, 2350 or 40% were selected because of raised lipid levels and 3449 or 58% were randomly selected.

Baseline data for the current analyses were obtained at visit 2. The visit 2 examination included fasting determinations of plasma lipids and lipoproteins, a physical examination, resting and stress electrocardiograms, and an in depth interview which included questions on personal habits such as current cigarette smoking and alcohol consumption. Women were also asked about their reproductive and menstrual histories.

Oestrogen use was determined by asking women if they had taken oral contraceptives or oestrogens within the 2 weeks before visit 2. For purposes of validation, participants were requested to bring samples and drug containers with them to the interview. The trade or generic name of each medication used was recorded. Colour illustrations of common medications and telephone calls to physicians and pharmacists were used to help identify drugs. Non-contraceptive oestrogen use was validated in 95% of women included as oestrogen users in this study. Over two-thirds of the women reporting oestrogen use were using premarin (natural conjugated oestrogens). Only 5 (1%) oestrogen users were also taking progestins.

All white women 30 years of age and older at visit 2 were included in a mortality follow-up study. The vital status of each participant, determined at each clinic annually, is currently known for over 99% of the cohort. When a person is identified as deceased, the local clinic coordinator requests a copy of the death certificate. The clinic physician reviews all death certificates before forwarding them to the LRC Central Patient Registry for coding by a nosologist (8th revision of the International Classification of Diseases). If there is any mention of CVD on the death certificate, the clinic data coordinator requests copies of all hospital and physician records (if a hospital or physician visit occurred within 30 days of death) and obtains an interview with the deceased's next-of-kin. All information regarding the death (for example, hospital records, physician records, personal interviews) is then forwarded to the Central Patient Registry.

These records are then blinded and reviewed independently for classification of the cause of death by two cardiologists who are members of the LRC Mortality Classification Panel. A standard algorithm is used for classification. If the two cardiologists do not agree about the specific cause of death the classification is adjudicated by the full panel of five cardiologists. In these analyses, death was considered as being caused by CVD if so defined by the LRC Mortality Classification Panel.

The present study was restricted to the 2389 white women aged 40–69 years at visit 2. Women who reported using oral contraceptives (n=91) or who had lacked information about menstrual status (n=29) or oestrogen use (n=1) were excluded, resulting in a final sample of 2269 women.

CVD death rates were based on numbers of deaths, age at death and person-years of observation. Women were followed for an average of 6.6 years, and persons aged 60–69 at visit 2 could therefore contribute person-years and events in the 70–79 years category. CVD death rates were age-adjusted by the indirect method using CVD (ICD 390–448) death rates from the 1976 US white female population as the standard.[37,38] 95% confidence limits on the relative risk were calculated.[39] The Cox proportional hazards model[40] was used to assess the independent effect of oestrogen use after adjustment for the standard CVD risk factors (age, blood pressure, cholesterol, smoking).

Women with CVD at visit 2 were defined as including those who: (1) reported a history of myocardial infarction (MI) or stroke; (2) reported use of medication for angina pectoris, or who had a Rose questionnaire diagnosis of angina, or treadmill angina; (3) reported using antiarrhythmic agents or digitalis or propranolol; (4)

136

were excluded from the treadmill test because of congestive heart failure, R-on-T type premature ventricular contractions, ventricular tachycardia, parasystolic focus, atrial flutter, or atrial fibrillation; or (5) had diagnostic or equivocal ECG evidence of MI.

RESULTS

Previous analysis after 5.6 years follow-up in this cohort[41] showed that women who were using oestrogens at visit 2 had a significantly lower risk of death from all causes (relative risk=0.37) than women not using oestrogens. This present analysis, based on additional events and person-years of follow-up, confirms the previous finding. After 6.6 years' follow-up oestrogen users still had a significantly lower risk of death from all causes than non-users (relative risk = 0.39).

The age-specific and age-adjusted CVD death rates for oestrogen users and non-users are presented in Table 11.4. There was a total of 34 CVD deaths in oestrogen non-users (total deaths=77; total non-users=1676) and only four CVD deaths in oestrogen users (total deaths=13; total users=593). At every age, oestrogen users had lower CVD rates than non-users. After adjustment for age, the relative risk of CVD mortality in users compared with non-users was 0.30 (95% confidence limits=0.08 to 0.91).

The relative difference in CVD rates in oestrogen users compared with non-users might be due to abnormally high death rates in the non-users, rather than lower rates in users. To address this possibility, standard mortality ratios (SMR) were calculated separately for oestrogen users and non-users. In non-users, the SMR was less than unity (SMR=0.76), although not significantly so. This result is consistent with the 'healthy participant' effect frequently observed in population-based studies. In users, however, the SMR was significantly less than 1.00 (SMR=0.22).

The Cox proportional hazards model was used to assess the effect of oestrogen use on CVD mortality while controlling for the standard CVD risk factors (Table 11.5). After statistical adjustment for age, systolic blood pressure, cholesterol, and

Table 11.4 CVD death rates (per 10 000) by age and oestrogen use.

Age (years)	User (n=593)	Non-user (n=1676)
40–49	0.0	0.0
	(0)*	(0)*
50–59	5.5	19.0
	(1)	(8)
60–69	8.1	46.3
	(1)	(14)
70–79	67.8	159.6
	(2)	(12)
Total	10.1	30.9
	(4)	(34)
Age-adjusted rate	12.2	41.8
Relative risk	0.30**	

* (number of deaths)
**95% confidence limits =0.09 to 0.91

Table 11.5 Cox model results. Multivariate association of standard CVD risk factors and oestrogen use with CVD death. CVD deaths=38.

Independent variables	β	SE of β	β/SE	Two-tailed p value
Age	0.140	0.028	5.07	0.000
Systolic blood pressure	0.016	0.006	2.45	0.014
Smoking	0.039	0.013	2.97	0.003
Total cholesterol	0.004	0.002	2.10	0.031
Oestrogen use	-1.033	0.532	1.94	0.052

SE=standard error

cigarette smoking, oestrogen use at baseline was negatively associated with CVD mortality ($\beta = -1.03$, two-tailed p = 0.052).

Because oestrogen use may have been avoided by women who were at high risk of CVD, additional analyses were done to ascertain whether the observed results could have been due to selection bias for oestrogen use. The prevalence of CVD at baseline in oestrogen users and non-users is presented in Table 11.6. The actual prevalence of CVD at visit 2 is somewhat higher in oestrogen users (13%) than in non-users (10%), due primarily to an excess of angina in users.

Table 11.6 Prevalence of CVD at baseline by oestrogen use.

Type of CVD	User (n=593)	Non-user (n=1676)
Angina medication only	0.5% (3)*	0.2% (4)*
ECG changes or Rose questionnaire angina	8.9% (53)	6.2. (104)
History of MI or stroke	4.5% (23)	4.0% (61)
All prevalent CVD	13.3% (79)	10.1% (169)

* (number of cases)

The prevalence of selected CVD medication use at baseline for oestrogen users and non-users is presented in Table 11.7. The consumption of the selected CVD medications was also somewhat higher in oestrogen users although, with the exception of blood pressure medication, the use of these drugs in this cohort is low.

There were also no differences between users and non-users by selection reason for visit 2. 42% of oestrogen users compared with 39% of non-users were selected in to the study because of raised lipid levels.

CVD rates were recalculated for oestrogen users and non-users after the exclusion of all women with prevalent CVD at baseline (Table 11.8). The resultant relative risk in users was 0.36 (confidence limits=0.07–1.22). Oestrogen used appeared to be protective both in women with prevalent CVD and in those free of disease at baseline. An additional Cox model with oestrogen use, age, smoking, blood pressure, and cholesterol was computed only for those women free of CVD at baseline. In this model, oestrogen use remained negatively associated with CVD mortality (estimated relative risk=0.35, p=0.09).

As oestrogens could have been avoided in women with a positive family history of

Table 11.7 Prevalence of selected CVD medication use by oestrogen at baseline.

CVD medication	Oestrogen user (n=593)	Oestrogen non-user (n=1676)
Antihypertensives	15.3%	12.2%
	(91)*	(204)*
Diuretics	15.5%	10.1%
	(92)	(169)
Angina medication	2.2%	1.5%
	(13)	(25)
Blood thinners	0.7%	0.7%
	(4)	(11)
Digitalis	0.7%	1.7%
	(4)	(28)
Antiarrhythmics	1.7%	1.1%
	(10)	(18)
Gout medication	1.7%	1.1%
	(10)	(19)
Diabetic agents	1.1%	2.3%
	(7)	(38)

* (number)

CVD, the reported prevalence of CVD in first-degree relatives of oestrogen users and non-users was compared. There were no differences between reported family history of CVD in oestrogen users and non-users, as 54% of users and 56% of non-users reported a paternal history of CVD, and 66% of users and 62% of non-users reported a maternal history of CVD.

A history of cigarette smoking was common among those women who died from CVD. Three of the four oestrogen users who died from CVD were smoking at visit 2 and one was an ex-smoker. Among the 34 deaths in non-users of oestrogen, 14 were smoking at visit 2, 12 were former smokers, and eight were women who had never smoked. When CVD death rates were recalculated separately for smokers and non-smokers, oestrogen use was negatively associated with CVD mortality in all smoking groups. The CVD death rate in oestrogen users who smoked was 23.1/10 000 compared with a rate of 40.7/10 000 in non-users who smoked. There were no CVD deaths among non-smoking oestrogen users, and the CVD mortality rate among non-smoking non-users was 14.4/10 000.

CVD death rates were also calculated separately for women with less than a high school education, high school graduates, and for those with at least some post-high school education. At each educational standard, oestrogen users had lower CVD rates (per 10 000) than non-users (0 vs 45.9; 16.7 vs 26.1; and 6.3 vs 25.6). Cox model analysis showed that educational standard did not alter the oestrogen-CVD mortality association.

Table 11.8 CVD mortality rates (per 10 000) by prevalence of CVD and oestrogen use at baseline.

Prevalent CVD	User	Non-user
No	8.5	23.8
	(3)*	(24)*
Yes	20.9	95.8
	(1)	(10)

* (number of deaths)

The potential confounding effects of exercise habits, body mass, menopausal status, and type of menopause (natural, surgical), were also examined in these analyses. However, none of these factors altered the mortality advantage of oestrogen users. The lower risk of CVD mortality in oestrogen users was also consistently seen in the individual LRC clinics.

As noted previously, exogenous oestrogen use increases HDL levels and decreases LDL levels. High levels of HDL are known to protect against the development of CVD and low levels of LDL are also known to be beneficial. Because of the lipoprotein changes in oestrogen users, we explored the possibility that the apparent protective effect of oestrogen use seen here was mediated through increased levels of HDL or decreased levels of LDL. The initial multivariable model (Table 11.5) included total cholesterol and not the lipoprotein fractions. In this first model the β coefficient for oestrogen was -1.03 and the p value$=0.052$. In a second model (Table 11.9) both HDL and LDL were substituted for total cholesterol along with oestrogen use, age, smoking, and blood pressure. In this second model, the association of oestrogen use with CVD mortality was substantially reduced as the size of the coefficient for oestrogen use was diminished by about 50% ($\beta=-0.559$, p$=0.30$). Regarding lipoprotein levels, HDL but not LDL was significantly associated with CVD mortality. Because of the small number of CVD deaths in the users, more definitive multivariate analysis on the complex association of oestrogen use, HDL, and CVD mortality could not be done. Additional multivariate analyses with other lipids and lipoproteins (triglycerides, VLDL) did not alter the association between oestrogen use and CVD mortality.

Table 11.9 Cox model results. Multivariate association of lipoproteins, other CVD risk factors, and oestrogen use with CVD death. CVD deaths$=38$.

Independent variables	β	SE of β	β/ SE	p value
Age	0.151	0.028	5.46	0.000
Systolic blood pressure	0.016	0.007	2.41	0.017
Smoking	0.041	0.013	3.10	0.002
LDC	0.004	0.003	1.21	0.225
HDC	-0.062	0.013	4.83	0.000
Oestrogen use	-0.520	0.542	0.96	0.338

SE=standard error

DISCUSSION

Oestrogens

The results presented here suggest that exogenous oestrogen use during the menopause may be protective against the development of fatal CVD. In this study, women using oestrogens at baseline had a significantly lower risk of fatal CVD during a 6.6 year follow-up period than non-users. Differences between users and non-users with regard to age, cigarette smoking, total cholesterol and blood pressure did not account for the lower risk of CVD mortality in users.

As oestrogens may not have been prescribed, or may have been discontinued in women who were at an increased risk of CVD, additional analyses were done to identify possible selection biases for oestrogen use. Because of the purposes of the LRC Program (including the identification of factors associated with CVD), careful and comprehensive evaluations of CVD status in all participants were done at baseline. Our results show that women reporting oestrogen use, compared with those not using oestrogens, were slightly more likely to have CVD at visit 2 (13% vs 10%). Essentially there were no differences between users and non-users in the occurrence of family history of CVD, CVD medication consumption, and selection reason to visit 2 (random vs increased lipids). Given these results, it seems unlikely that users were selected for oestrogen use because they had less CVD than non-users.

The possibility was considered that CVD death rates in non-users are exceptionally high, rather than exceptionally low among users. This situation could lead to an apparent protective effect in oestrogen users. When compared with an external standard (US rates), however, oestrogen users have a significantly lower CVD mortality than expected (SMR=0.22), while the CVD death rate in non-users is lower than unity (SMR=0.76), but significantly so. These findings support the hypothesis that the CVD mortality difference between users and non-users in our study is due to the low CVD mortality rates among users.

Another interpretation of the results presented here is that oestrogen use is protective against death from CVD only in women with CVD. To test this hypothesis, we excluded from the analysis all women with CVD at visit 2. After exclusion of all prevalent cases, the relative risk of CVD death in users compared with non-users was 0.36 (95% confidence limits=0.07–1.22). In addition, in both women with and without prevalent CVD at visit 2, oestrogen users had lower CVD rates than non-users. Finally, adjustment for the major CVD risk factors via the multivariate model in women free of CVD at baseline did not appreciably alter the negative association of oestrogen use with CVD mortality ($\beta=-1.037$, p=0.09).

The results of this study must be reconciled with those of other studies which suggest that oestrogen use increases the risk of CVD rather than protects against CVD. Several of the earlier studies in which oestrogens were found to increase the risk of CVD were conducted in men rather than women.[9-12] As noted previously, the doses of oestrogen given to these men tended to be rather high, certainly much higher than that routinely prescribed today for replacement therapy in women.[42] Furthermore, the more potent synthetic oestrogens (ethinyloestradiol, DES) rather than natural oestrogens were frequently used. In addition, all of the studies in men were either CVD secondary prevention trials[9,10] or in much older men with prostatic cancer.[11,12] Given that oestrogens may have different effects in women than in men, and given that the men evaluated in these trials were older, sick, and given higher doses than usually prescribed for menopausal symptoms, it seems inappropriate to generalise these findings to menopausal women.

Oral contraceptives
The other substantial and consistent evidence which suggests that oestrogens increase the risk of CVD comes from studies of oral contraceptive users. Oestrogens prescribed for menopausal symptoms are not, however, the same drugs as those

used for contraceptive purposes in younger women. The menopausal oestrogens most commonly prescribed are natural conjugated oestrogens, and these are prescribed at a relatively low dose (0.3–1.25 mg/day). These oestrogens have been shown to increase HDL and decrease LDL levels.[8,43–45] On the other hand, the oral contraceptives used by younger women are usually combinations of more potent synthetic oestrogens and progestins and are prescribed in higher doses than menopausal oestrogens. The association of increased CVD mortality in oral contraceptive users has been attributed to their oestrogenic content, although recently it has been suggested that progestins and the progestin components of oral contraceptives may be related to the risk of disease.[8,33] And, unlike menopausal oestrogens, the effect of oral contraceptives on lipid/lipoprotein levels may be detrimental, as progestins have been shown to increase LDL levels.[8,46] Given the differences (in potency, dose, and agents) between oestrogens and oral contraceptives, it also seems inappropriate to claim that oestrogens increase the risk of CVD based on the oral contraceptive experience.

Those results showing a significantly increased CVD risk in menopausal oestrogen users are found in four reports [30–32,35] from only two study populations. In data from the Framingham study,[33] the excess occurrence of CVD in users appears to be primarily from angina (relative risk=2.3), a relatively soft endpoint, although there is an increased risk for all other manifestations of coronary heart disease (relative risk=1.6). The risks for oestrogen users of 7.5 and 9.3 reported by Jick et al [31,32] seem excessive given the magnitude of the other risks reported. These studies also had small numbers of cases, a low proportion of participation from both cases and controls, and a high proportion of smokers (94%) among the cases.

Overall most studies of menopausal oestrogen use in women purportedly show no positive association between oestrogen use and CVD risk; [26–29,33,34] however, many of the actual risks presented (either overall, or for selected subgroups) are less than one. [26–29] In several of these studies [27,28,33,34] only a small proportion of cases were using oestrogens; hence the power to detect any oestrogenic effects may have been low.

Results
Our findings suggest that oestrogen users have about one-third the occurrence of fatal CVD of non-users. This risk estimate is similar to those estimates from the other studies which show a significant protective effect of oestrogen use.[22–25]

These differing results from a variety of studies of menopausal oestrogen in women may partially be explained by differences in methodologies, endpoints, or age groups of women under study. For example, those reports, including this one, which show a protective effect of oestrogen use [22,24,25] tend to have fatal CVD events as the outcome of interest while those showing an increased risk tend to examine only non-fatal events. [30–32,34,35] Likewise, the studies which show a protective effect tend to examine middle-aged women (>45 years), while those showing an increased risk in users tend to be looking at younger women (> 45 years). Finally, those studies which showed a very high risk to oestrogen users [31,32] had serious methodological problems due to a low participation rate and potential confounding by smoking. In summary, none of the studies presented here, including this one, is without limitations.

In this study we do not have complete information on the type, dosage, or duration of oestrogen used. This limits our understanding in that we cannot assess whether a dose-response, or duration-of-use effect is present.

As in most prospective studies, exposure (oestrogen use) was ascertained at only one point in time, and therefore users and non-users may have either quit or begun oestrogen use during the follow-up interval. The effect of these potential misclassifications, however, should bias our results towards one. That is, if oestrogen use 'truly' protects against CVD death, then inclusion of past or subsequent users in the non-user group would tend to reduce the death rate in non-users—that is, the true CVD mortality in the non-user group would be higher than that observed here. Classifying women who subsequently stopped using oestrogens as users would tend to increase the death rate seen in the user group. Thus the true difference in mortality between oestrogen users and non-users may be even larger than we observed, and our results would be an underestimation of the true relative risk. If oestrogen has no effect on CVD mortality, then classification would not affect the results. And finally, if oestrogen use actually increases the risk of CVD death, the likelihood of observing a statistically significantly lower CVD risk in users (as was seen in this study) is extremely small.

As in most observational studies, we have no knowledge about why a woman was or was not prescribed oestrogens. The possibility exists that despite the similar CVD profile seen in users and non-users, women who are prescribed these drugs are different from non-users in some as yet undefined but confounding way. If this is indeed the case, then it is of great importance to identify any factors which might account for this, given the marked reduction in CVD mortality in users.

In conclusion, in a population-based cohort of women followed for an average of 6.6 years, those reporting oestrogen use at baseline had a significantly lower risk of CVD death than non-users. Given the magnitude of the problem of CVD in women, the high prevalence of oestrogen use, and ambiguous and conflicting study results, additional studies of postmenopausal oestrogen use and CVD in women are urgently needed.

SUMMARY

Do postmenopausal oestrogens influence the risk of cardiovascular disease (CVD) in women? To address this question, a total of 2269 white women aged 40–69 years of age were followed prospectively in the Lipid Research Clinics Program Follow-Up Study. After an average follow-up period of 6.6 years, women using oestrogens at baseline had a significantly lower risk of death from CVD than women not using oestrogens (relative risk=0.30). Multivariable adjustment for the standard cardiovascular risk factors (age, smoking, blood pressure and cholesterol levels) did not alter the mortality advantage seen in oestrogen users (estimated relative risk=0.36). Additional analyses to discover whether selection bias for oestrogen use might have influenced the findings showed no significant differences between oestrogen users and non-users. A protective effect of oestrogen use is biologically plausible because oestrogens increase high-density lipoprotein (HDL) cholesterol, and high levels of HDL are known to protect against CVD. Further multivariate analyses in this cohort suggest that increased HDL levels among oestrogen users explained a substantial proportion of their lower cardiovascular death rate.

REFERENCES

[1]Stadel BV, Weiss N. Characteristics of menopausal women: a survey of King and Pierce counties in Washington, 1973-1974. Am J Epidemiol 1975; 102: 209–16.

[2]Pfeffer RI. Estrogen use in postmenopausal women. Am J Epidemiol 1977; 105: 21–9.

[3]Ajabor LN, Tsai CC, Vela P, Yen SSC. Effect of exogenous estrogen on carbohydrate metabolism in postmenopausal women. Am J Obstet Gynecol 1972; 113: 383–7.

[4]Coope J, Thomson JM, Poller L. Effects of 'natural oestrogen' replacement therapy on menopausal symptoms and blood clotting. Br Med J 1975; 4: 139–43.

[5]Bonnar J, Haddon M, Hunter DH, Richards DH, Thornton C. Coagulation system changes in post-menopausal women receiving oestrogen preparations. Postgrad Med J 1976; 52(suppl 6): 30–4.

[6]Wallentin L, Larsson-Cohn U. Metabolic and hormonal effects of post-menopausal oestrogen replacement treatment. II. Plasma lipids. Acta Endocrinol (Kbh) 1977; 86: 597–607.

[7]Silfverstolpe G, Gustafson A, Samsioe G, Svanborg A. Lipid metabolic studies in oophorectomized women; effects induced by two different estrogens on serum lipids and lipoproteins. Gynecol Obstet Invest 1980; 11: 161–9.

[8]Wahl P, Walden C, Knopp R et al. Effects of estrogen/progestin potency on lipid/lipoprotein cholesterol. N Engl J Med 1983; 308: 862–7.

[9]The Coronary Drug Project Research Group. The Coronary Drug Project. Initial findings leading to modifications of its research protocol. JAMA 1970; 214: 1303–13.

[10]The Coronary Drug Project Research Group. The Coronary Drug Project. Findings leading to discontinuation of the 2.5 mg/day estrogen group. JAMA 1973; 226: 652–7.

[11]Blackard CE, Doe RP, Mellinger GT, Byar DP. Incidence of cardiovascular disease and death in patients receiving diethylstilbestrol for carcinoma of the prostate. Cancer 1970; 26: 249–56.

[12]Byar DP. The Veterans Administration Cooperative Urological Research Group's Studies of cancer of the prostate. Cancer 1973; 32: 1126–30.

[13]Vessey MP, Doll R. Investigation of the relation between use of oral contraceptives and thromboembolic disease. Br Med J 1968; 2: 199–205.

[14]Sartwell PE, Masi AT, Arthes FG et al. Thromboembolism and oral contraceptives: an epidemiologic case-control study. Am J Epidemiol 1969; 90: 365–80.

[15]Inman WHW, Vessey MP, Westerholm B, Engelund A. Thromboembolic disease and the steroidal content of oral contraceptives—a report to the committee on safety of drugs. Br Med J 1970; 2: 203–9.

[17]Pick R, Stamler J, Rodbard S, Katz LN. Inhibition of coronary atherosclerosis by estrogens in cholesterol-fed chicks. Circulation 1952; 6: 276–80.

[18]Pick R, Stamler J, Rodbard S, Katz LN. Estrogen-induced regression of coronary atherosclerosis in cholesterol-fed chicks. Circulation 1952; 6: 858–61.

[19]Robinson RW, Higano N, Cohen WD. Increased incidence of coronary heart disease in women castrated prior to the menopause. Arch Intern Med 1959; 104: 908–13.

[20]Parrish HM, Carr CA, Hall DG et al. Time interval from castration in premenopausal women to development of excessive coronary atherosclerosis. Am J. Obstet Gynecol 1967; 99: 155–62.

[21]Rivin AU, Dimitroff SP. The incidence and severity of atherosclerosis in estrogen-treated males, and in females with a hypoestrogenic or a hyperestrogenic state. Circulation 1954; 9: 533–9.

[22]Burch JC, Byrd BF Jr, Vaughn WK. The effects of long-term estrogen on hysterectomized women. Am J Obstet Gynecol 1974; 118: 778–82.

[23]Hammond CB, Jelovsek FR, Lee KL, Greasman WT, Parker RT. Effects of long-term estrogen replacement therapy. 1. Metabolic effects. Am J Obstet Gynecol 1979; 133: 525–36.

[24]Nachtigall LE, Nachtigall RH, Nachtigall RD, Beckman EM. Estrogen replacement therapy II: a prospective study in the relationship to carcinoma and cardiovascular and metabolic problems. Obstet Gynecol 1979; 54: 74–9.

[25]Ross RK, Paganini-Hill A, Mack TM, Arthur M, Henderson BE. Menopausal oestrogen therapy and protection from death from ischaemic heart disease. Lancet 1981; 1: 858–60.

[26]Pfeffer RI, Whipple GH, Kurosaki TT, Chapman JM. Coronary risk and estrogen therapy in postmenopausal women. N Engl J Med 1976; 294: 1256–9.

[27]Rosenberg L, Armstrong B, Phil D, Jick HJ. Myocardial infarction and estrogen therapy in post-menopausal women. N Engl J Med 1976; 294: 1256–9.

[28]Adams S, Williams V, Vessey MP. Cardiovascular disease and hormone replacement treatment: a pilot case-control study. Br Med J 1981; 282: 1277-8.

[29]Bain C, Willett W, Hennekens CH, Rosner B, Belanger C, Speizer FE. Use of postmenopausal hormones and risk of myocardial infarction. Circulation 1981; 64: 42-6.

[30]Gordon T, Kannel WB, Hjortland MC, McNamara PM. Menopause and coronary heart disease—the Framingham Study. Ann Intern Med 1978; 89: 157-61.

[31]Jick H, Dinan B, Rothman KJ. Noncontraceptive estrogens and nonfatal myocardial infarction. JAMA 1978; 239: 1407-8.

[32]Jick H, Dinan B, Herman R, Rothman KJ. Myocardial infarction and other vascular diseases in young women. JAMA 1978; 240: 2548-52.

[33]Petitti DB, Wingerd J, Pellegrin F, Ramcharan S. Risk of vascular disease in women: smoking, oral contraceptives, noncontraceptive estrogens, and other factors. JAMA 1979; 242: 1150-4.

[34]Rosenberg L, Slone D, Shapiro S, Kaufman D, Stalley PD, Miettinen OS. Noncontraceptive estrogens and myocardial infarction in young women. JAMA 1980; 244: 339-42.

[35]Wilson PWF, Garrison RJ, Castelli WP. Postmenopausal estrogen use and cardiovascular morbidity: the Framingham Study. CVD Epidemiol Newslett 1984; 35: 35. (Abstract)

[36]The Lipid Research Clinics Epidemiology Committee. Plasma lipid distributions in selected North American populations: The Lipid Research Clinics Program Prevalence Study. Circulation 1979; 60: 427-39.

[37]Vital Statistics of the United States 1976: II. Mortality Part B, publication 79-1102. Washington, DC: US Dept of Health, Education, and Welfare, 1979.

[38]Vital Statistics of the United States: II. Mortality Part A, publication 80-1101. Washington, DC: US Dept of Health, Education, and Welfare, 1980.

[39]Ederer F, Mantel N. Confidence limits on the ratio of two Poisson variables. Am J Epidemiol 1974; 100: 165-7.

[40]Cox DR. Regression models and life-tables. J R Stat Soc B 1972; 34: 187-220.

[41]Bush TL, Cowan LD, Barrett-Connor E et al. Estrogen use and all-cause mortality. Preliminary results from the Lipid Research Clinics Program Follow-up Study. JAMA 1983; 249: 903-6.

[42]Hammond CB, Maxson WS. Current status of estrogen therapy for the menopause. Fertil Steril 1982; 37: 5-25.

[43]Issacs AJ, Harvard CWH. Effect of piperazine oestrone sulphate on serum lipids and lipoproteins in menopausal women. Acta Endocrinol 1977; 85: 143-50.

[44]Bradley DD, Wingerd J, Petitti DB, Kraus RM, Ramcharan S. Serum high-density-lipoprotein cholesterol in women using oral contraceptives, estrogens and progestins. N Engl J Med 1978; 299: 17-20.

[45]Wallace RB, Hoover J, Barrett-Connor E et al. Altered plasma lipid and lipoprotein levels associat ed with oral contraceptive and oestrogen use: report from the Medications Working Group of the Lipid Research Clinics Program. Lancet 1979; 2: 111-5.

[46]Hirvonen E, Mälkönen M, Manninen V. Effects of different progestogens on lipoproteins during postmenopausal replacement therapy. N Engl J Med 1981; 304: 560-3.

Discussion on Chapter 11

Shapiro
I am in a difficult position. These data were presented at the American Society for Epidemiological Research in June 1983. I was asked to be the formal discussant of this presentation. I was very critical of the results, and I will try quickly to summarise why. There were several difficulties in this study which, in my view, raise questions of validity.

Oestrogen use was defined as any use during the 2 weeks before the second visit. That definition may have been adequate for evaluating lipoprotein patterns, but it was not adequate for evaluating subsequent cardiovascular mortality trends. There was no information on exposure before the myocardial infarction, none on shifts after initial classification into exposed or non-exposed groups, none on duration of use, none on the prevalence on previous use—either among those initially classified as exposed or those initially classified as non-exposed. It is difficult to understand why this information is not available, because it would have been obtained when subsequent questionnaires were sent out. Dr Rifkind has referred to the misclassification of the exposed tending to obscure the effect so that the real effect would be even stronger. The argument is true in principle, but the corollary is also true—namely, that when there is substantial misclassification there is a substantial opportunity for bias.

There were also other problems. One was that in a longitudinal study it might be expected that younger women who were not yet menopausal and not on oestrogens would, as they aged and reached the menopause, come on to oestrogens. Similarly, it might be expected that older women at the time of menopause would continue on oestrogens and then tend to stop as they aged. Hence, oestrogen exposure status at the time of the myocardial infarction was not available.

A further difficulty is that the data were exceedingly sparse. There were four cases of cardiovascular disease in the oestrogen-exposed, one of whom had a pulmonary embolism and one of whom had cardiac failure. Only two had myocardial infarction—which is the relevant outcome. There was a corresponding reduction in numbers among the non-exposed women. The number of cases of infarction in both the exposed and the non-exposed were insufficient to justify any conclusion.

Another difficulty is that earlier on, the investigators had suggested that oestrogens reduce all-cause mortality. There is really no plausible biological mechanism. If one subtracts the cardiovascular mortality and looks at mortality in the women who died of non-cardiovascular causes, the crude relative risk estimate is 0.5. That is a result that could be due to chance; but, if it is not, it will be due to a systematic error which may or may not be identified. If it cannot be identified, it may be that if the oestrogen users were analogous to Mormons or Seventh Day Adventists—perhaps they would have a reduced all-cause mortality. It could be that oestrogen users, like these groups, take the trouble to take better care of themselves. In any event when a cohort study has only some 500 exposed, when it uses a definition of exposure based on a point prevalence of 2 weeks' oestrogen use, and when it ends up with only two cases of myocardial infarction. I cannot agree that this provides informative evidence suggestive of a reduction in the risk of myocardial infarction attributable to oestrogen use.

Rifkind
I hope I made clear during the presentation that we were not claiming that we had established the facts beyond doubt. However, given the strength of the observations we felt bound to report the findings and to take some account of them in the context of the other work on this topic. I will not attempt to respond to all the issues but only to a few points. Although there is a small number of oestrogen users, there is a much larger number in the non-user group. In a sense we are the victims of the markedly reduced relative risk. Details are available on the various categories of cardiovascular risk. Although the number of cases with cardiovascular disease is indeed relatively small the analyses showed statistical significance. Another reason for reassurance, even with the relatively small numbers, is that the conventional risk factors were operating—age, cigarette smoking, blood pressure, total plasma cholesterol and HDL cholesterol levels—which reflected their relationships to risk.

Wilhelmsson
Do you know anything about differences in social class between women taking or not taking oral contraceptives? According to some studies low social class is associated with increased risk for myocardial infarction.

Rifkind
We looked at several factors, among them education, as an index of social class, and they did not confound the findings.

Beaumont
What type of oestrogen treatment did the women take?

Rifkind
About 70% of the women reported using premarin.

Oliver
Is it conceivable that the users had a lower cigarette smoking habit than the non-users? On the assumption that doctors should know that it is a bad thing to give an oestrogen to people who smoke, they are more likely to give it to those who don't smoke. Have you got a relatively low-risk group on the basis of low cigarette smoking habits? I did notice in your Cox regression model that the cigarettes were at 0.002—a level very similar in view of the small numbers that you have for HDL.

Rifkind
The Cox model showed that cigarette smoking is an independent and powerful predictor of subsequent cardiovascular disease. It also showed that, when adjustment is made for cigarette smoking, oestrogen use still retains an independent predictive power. Further, in a simpler analysis which looks at the relative risk for oestrogen users and non-users who are either cigarette smokers or non-smokers, the relative risk is reduced in each category of oestrogen user.

Oliver
Those numbers must be small. I wonder if I might ask a different question of the Framingham people. Would they comment on the preliminary announcement made recently by them which concerns the use of postmenopausal oestrogen and cardiovascular mortality—which, I understand, is mostly angina. In spite of a more favourable initial cardiovascular risk profile, after control for major known risk factors women who reported usage of postmenopausal oestrogens in the 12 year study showed a greater than 50% increased rate for cardiovascular morbidity at the 1% level of significance. In other words, the opposite of what we have just heard. Would somebody comment on this?

Rifkind
I did mention the Framingham study as one of the several cohort studies with findings that appear to be contrary to those of the Lipid Research Clinics. One can speculate on different preparations or the use of different endpoints.

Haynes
When the Framingham data were presented in March 1983 at the American Heart Association Council on Epidemiology meetings Dr Peter Wilson showed that oestrogen use was only significantly related to the incidence in angina pectoris. The other finding observed was an inverse association of relative weight with subsequent disease in that same group of women—that is, being thin is associated with coronary heart disease in the Framingham women. A hypothesis follows this finding: women may take postmenopausal oestrogens if they are depressed; since depression is related to poor appetite—and subsequently thin people—then depression may have been the real cause of the association in the Framingham data rather than the use of postmenopausal oestrogens.

Angina is the strongest disease outcome on the oestrogen study. There may be some confounding in terms of the economic status of the women in Framingham and the women in the Lipid Research Clinics population project. The older women basically came from two clinics: the Lajolla clinic, which included upper-class white women, and the Oklahoma clinic which included middle-class white women. A few older women scattered throughout the rest of the clinics were also included, so the LRC population is not dealing with a lower-class group of women. In Framingham, on the other hand, there were more blue-collar working women, 80% of them working in clerical or blue-collar jobs. 50% of these women worked outside the home. Thus the difference in the LRC and Framingham studies might also be due to the types of women in the populations.

Wynn
May I ask you Dr Rifkind about your use of postmenopausal oestrogen? Do you really mean oestrogen, or is progestogen used in the regimen?

Rifkind
About 1% of the women reported the use of a preparation containing progestin.

Wynn
If your data are valid, I think that as far as cardiovascular disease is concerned there

is an implication that it is the progestogen which is dangerous in the oral contraceptive and not the oestrogen. Would you agree with that?

Rifkind

I think so. Much of the focus and publicity on oestrogen use has been on endometrial cancer. The rate of endometrial cancer is relatively small. For example, in our study to date there has been no case of endometrial cancer. We may be seeing a movement away from using oestrogens alone—which might have widespread cardiovascular benefit—to avoid a much less common condition.

Shapiro

We have data that suggest that long-term oestrogen use continues to convey an increased risk of endometrial cancer for several years after use. It could be that you failed to observe an association because you used a short-term definition of exposure. The incidence of endometrial cancer is not all that low—about half that of breast cancer.

Rifkind

Its contribution to mortality is less than its non-fatal prevalence.

12. The relation between myocardial infarction and cigarette smoking in women under 50 years of age: modifying influence of individual risk factors

L. Rosenberg

Cigarette smoking may be related to as much as two-thirds of the incidence of first myocardial infarctions (MI) in women under 50 years of age.[1-3] We have previously assessed the influence of an underlying predisposition to an infarction on the association between risk and smoking, but numbers were too small to examine the effects of specific predisposing factors.[3] In the present report, based on a larger series, we evaluate separately the effects of several major risk factors for MI on the association between MI and cigarette smoking.

SUBJECTS AND METHODS

This report is based on a case-control study of first non-fatal MI in relation to oral contraceptive use in women under 50 years of age.[4,5] The data were collected in two phases: in the first,[4] women admitted to hospital for first MIs (cases)[6] and women admitted for conditions thought to be unrelated to oral contraceptive use (controls) were interviewed in hospital; in the second,[5] further information was collected from selected participants in their homes and a blood sample was drawn.

Data collection
In phase 1, conducted from 1976–79, cases and controls were interviewed in 155 hospitals located in the metropolitan areas of Boston, New York, and Philadelphia; the refusal rate was 5%.[4] Information was obtained by standard questionnaire on personal characteristics and habits (including cigarette smoking), medical history, and drug use. After excluding women with unknown smoking habits, 554 cases and 2005 controls remained. The controls were group-matched to the cases within 5 year age groups in a ratio of 4:1, except at age 45–49 where the ratio was 3.4:1. The women aged 25–49 years of age and none had a history of previous MI. The median age in both the cases and the controls was 44 years. In the controls, who had been admitted for fractures and sprains, orthopaedic disorders, infections and a variety of other conditions, smoking habits were similar across the diagnostic categories.[2]

In phase 2, conducted from 1978–81, cases from the first phase who lived in areas chosen for accessibility were visited in their homes; about three controls per case in the same areas were also visited.[5] The refusal rate was 14% among eligible cases and

27% among eligible controls. Blood samples were drawn for determination of ABO blood group and lipoprotein analysis, and information was obtained on history of MI or stroke before age 60 in a parent or sibling. In addition, a 10-question personality questionnaire, designed to measure time-urgency and competitiveness, was administered. There were 254 cases, among whom the median age was 44 years, and 794 controls, among whom the median age was 42 years.

Analysis
Relative risk estimates were aggregated across strata by the Mantel-Haenszel procedure,[7] and 95% confidence intervals were calculated by Miettinen's method.[8] Relative risk estimates given in this report were adjusted for age only (25–39, 40–44, 45–49), since allowance for other factors changed the estimates very little.

In the tables that follow there are variations in the totals because of the exclusion of subjects, with unknown values for particular factors, and because some information was obtained only from the participants in phase 2.

Potential bias
To assess whether participation in phase 2 had been conditional on smoking, we compared the smoking habits of phase 1 and phase 2 participants. They were similar. Among cases, the proportion who were non-smokers was 19% in phase 1 and 17% in phase 2, and 48% and 55%, respectively, smoked 25 or more cigarettes a day. Among controls, the proportion of non-smokers in phase 1 was 45% and in phase 2 it was 47%; 19% and 20%, respectively, smoked 25 or more cigarettes a day.

RESULTS

Among the 554 cases, 81% were current smokers (in the year before admission), compared with 55% of the 2005 controls (Table 12.1). The estimated relative risk of MI for smokers compared with women who had never smoked increased with the number of cigarettes smoked per day, from 1.4 for the lightest smokers (less than 15

Table 12.1 Cigarette smoking in 554 cases and 2005 controls.

		Never smoked	Ex-smoker	Current smoker * (cig/day)			
				1–14	15–24	25–34	≥35
Cases	No	73	35	40	139	96	171
	(%)	(13)	(6)	(7)	(25)	(17)	(31)
Controls	No	616	280	241	496	166	206
	(%)	(31)	(14)	(12)	(25)	(8)	(10)
Relative risk estimate +		1.0**	1.0	1.4	2.4	5.0	7.0
95% confidence interval				0.7–1.6	0.9–2.1	1.8–3.3	3.6–6.9	5.2–9.4

* Last smoked at least 1 year before admission
** Reference category
+ Allowance made for age (25–39, 40–44, 45–49)

Table 12.2 Cigarette smoking in 554 cases and 2005 controls, by age.

Age (years)		Never smoked	Ex-smoker	Current smoker (cig/day)			
				1–14	15–24	25–34	≥35
25–39	Cases	10	5	4	25	23	41
	Controls	134	52	56	112	32	42
	Relative risk estimate	1.0*	1.3	1.0	3.0	9.6	13
40–44	Cases	18	4	8	40	28	58
	Controls	173	88	65	170	61	64
	Relative risk estimate	1.0*	0.4	1.2	2.3	4.4	8.7
45–49	Cases	45	26	28	74	45	72
	Controls	309	140	120	214	73	100
	Relative risk estimate	1.0*	1.3	1.6	2.4	4.2	4.9

* Reference category

cigarettes a day) to 7.0 for the heaviest (at least 35 cigarettes a day). For ex-smokers (who last smoked at least 1 year before admission) the relative risk estimate was 1.0.

The association of risk with the number of cigarettes smoked was apparent in each age group (Table 12.2), but the relative risk point estimates tended to be higher at younger ages: for the heaviest smokers relative to women who never smoked, the point estimate was 13 at 25–39 years of age, 8.7 at 40–44, and 4.9 at 45–49 ($p < 0.05$ for the difference between estimates in the youngest and oldest age groups).

Table 12.3 Cigarette smoking in 554 cases and 2005 controls, by oral contraceptive use*.

Oral contraceptive use		Non-smoker **	Current smoker(cig/day)	
			1–24	≥ 25
Current‡	Cases	3	6	32
	Controls	19	23	9
	Relative risk estimate†	(1.0)††	3.2	23
	95% confidence interval		0.5–22	6.8–87
Past	Cases	33	67	105
	Controls	320	285	146
	Relative risk estimate	(1.0)††	2.3	6.7
	95% confidence interval		1.5–3.6	4.5–10
Never	Cases	72	106	130
	Controls	557	429	217
	Relative risk estimate	(1.0)††	1.9	4.7
	95% confidence interval		1.4–2.7	3.4–6.5

* Data on oral contraceptive use collected in phase 1
** Women who never smoked and ex-smokers
† Allowance made for age (25–29, 30–34, 35–39, 40–44, 45–49)
†† Reference category
‡ Used within previous month

In Table 12.3, the smoking habits of the cases and controls are given according to categories of oral contraceptive use (data from phase 1). The risk of MI increased with the amount smoked in each category, but the point estimate of relative risk for smokers of 25 or more cigarettes a day was greater among women who were current users (within the previous month) (relative risk=23) than among women who had never used oral contraceptives (relative risk=4.7; p<0.05 for the difference) or among women who used them only in the past (relative risk = 7.7; p>0.05 for the difference). Women who were both current users of oral contraceptives and smokers of at least 25 cigarettes a day were estimated to have 23 times (95% confidence interval, 12–44) the risk of MI of non-smokers who never used the pill.

Table 12.4 Cigarette smoking in 254 cases and 794 controls by total plasma cholesterol level*.

Total plasma cholesterol (mmol/l)		Non-smoker**	Current smoker (cig/day) 1–24	≥ 25
<5.2	Cases	17	24	31
	Controls	194	126	84
	Relative risk estimate†	(1.0)††	2.4	4.2
	95% confidence interval		1.2–4.7	2.3–7.6
5.2–6.5	Cases	16	22	66
	Controls	139	96	57
	Relative risk estimate	(1.0)††	2.2	11
	95% confidence interval		1.1–4.3	6.0–20
> 6.5	Cases	9	27	41
	Controls	40	36	18
	Relative risk estimate	(1.0)††	3.3	9.9
	95% confidence interval		1.4–7.9	4.2–24

* Data on cholesterol collected in phase 2
**Women who never smoked and ex-smokers
† Allowance made for age (25–39, 40–44, 45–49)
††Reference category

As shown in Table 12.4, the association of MI risk with the amount smoked was present at low (<5.2 mmol/l), intermediate (5.2–6.4 mmol/l), and high (>6.5 mmol/l) levels of total plasma cholesterol (data on cholesterol from phase 2). Among women with levels less than 5.2 mmol/l, the estimated relative risk for smokers of 25 or more cigarettes daily, relative to non-smokers, was lower (relative risk=4.2) than that among women with intermediate levels (relative risk=11) or high levels (relative risk=4.2) than that among women with intermediate levels (relative risk=9.9), but only the differences between the estimate in the low and intermediate groups was statistically significant at the 0.05 level. Smokers of at least 25 cigarettes a day with total plasma cholesterol levels of at least 6.5 mmol/l were estimated to have a risk of MI 20 times (95% confidence interval, 11–27) that of non-smokers whose cholesterol levels were below 5.2 mmol/l.

In Table 12.5, the estimated relative risks of MI for smokers of at least 25 cigarettes a day relative to non-smokers are given according to several potential MI

Table 12.5 Smoking of at least 25 cigarettes a day in 554 cases and 2005 controls according to known and potential MI risk factors*.

Factor		Never smoked or ex-smoker Cases	Never smoked or ex-smoker Controls	Current smoker ≥ 25 cig/day Cases	Current smoker ≥ 25 cig/day Controls	Relative risk estimate**	95% confidence interval
History of treated	Yes	48	127	65	43	3.9	2.4–6.5
hypertension	No	60	767	199	329	7.9	5.9–11
History of treated angina	Yes	10	19	19	7	5.1	1.5–17
pectoris	No	96	862	240	357	6.1	4.7–7.9
History of treated diabetes	Yes	16	22	22	7	3.2	1.2–8.7
mellitus	No	91	869	245	364	6.6	5.1–8.5
Postmenopausal		35	338	65	159	3.9	2.5–6.1
Premenopausal		73	558	202	213	7.8	5.8–11
Body mass	≥ 40	44	272	74	89	5.6	3.6–8.6
index †	< 40	61	605	187	268	6.9	5.1–9.4

* Data on risk factors collected in phase 1
** Allowance made for age (25–39, 40–44, 45–49); reference category is non-smoking (never smoked or ex-smoker)
† 1b/in²×1000

Table 12.6 Smoking of at least 25 cigarettes a day in 254 cases and 794 controls according to known and potential MI risk factors*.

Factor		Never smoked or ex-smoker Cases	Never smoked or ex-smoker Controls	Current smoker ≥ 25 cig/day Cases	Current smoker ≥ 25 cig/day Controls	Relative risk estimate**	95% confidence interval
HDL cholesterol	< 40	28	94	75	64	4.2	2.4–7.2
mg/100 ml)	≥ 40	14	276	64	95	14	8.0–23
Blood group	A	20	144	66	53	10	5.7–17
	AB	3	48	11	26	9.4	2.4–38
	B	2	11	6	9	2.6	0.5–14
	O	17	172	56	71	8.1	4.6–14
Family history of MI or stroke before age 60	Present	18	119	61	57	7.2	4.0–13
	Absent	24	256	78	102	9.4	5.8–15
Personality score †	6.5–10.0	13	71	42	42	7.5	4.5–12
	0–6.4	29	297	96	116	10	5.7–18

* Data on risk factors collected in phase 2
** Allowance made for age (25–39, 40–44, 45–49); reference category is non-smoking (never smoked or ex-smoker)
† A higher score indicates a greater tendency to type A behaviour
HDL=high-density lipoprotein

risk factors on which information was collected in phase 1 (hypertension, angina pectoris, diabetes mellitus, menopausal status, and body mass index). Within each category of the risk factors examined, smoking was associated with an increased risk of MI. The magnitude of the relative risk tended to be smaller in women who had a particular risk factor (that is, who were at increased baseline risk of MI) than in women who did not. The relative risk estimate for smokers of at least 25 cigarettes a day among hypertensive women was 3.9, for example, compared with 7.9 among normotensive women.

Table 12.6 gives the relation of MI risk to smoking of at least 25 cigarettes a day according to several MI risk factors on which information was collected in phase 2 (high-density lipoprotein cholesterol, ABO blood group, family history of MI, and tendency to type A behaviour). Smoking was associated with an increased risk of MI within each category. Again, the relative increase in risk was generally smaller among women at higher baseline risk. The point estimates were slightly higher, however, among women with blood groups A or AB than among women with blood group O.

DISCUSSION

In this study of women under 50 years of age, the risk of MI increased with the number of cigarettes smoked. The relative increases in risk were similar in magnitude to those estimated by Mann et al[1] for non-fatal MI in young women and by Doll and Peto[9] for fatal ischaemic heart disease in young men. The association was apparent in each age group but was weaker in the older women, as expected.[9,10] In addition, among women predisposed to an infarction because of current oral contraceptive use, increased total cholesterol level, decreased high-density lipoprotein cholesterol level, hypertension, diabetes mellitus, angina pectoris, blood group A, tendency to type A behaviour, or family history of MI, the risk was increased still further by smoking. Clearly, the adverse effect of smoking occurs both in the presence and absence of the major risk factors for MI, and is not explicable by them.

In general, the relative increase in the risk associated with smoking was greater the lower the underlying level of risk. For example, at 45–49 years of age smokers of at least 35 cigarettes daily were estimated to have a risk of MI five times that of women who never smoked, while in women 25–39 years of age the corresponding increase was 13-fold. The absolute increase in risk attributable to smoking, however, would usually be greater among those whose baseline risk is high: this can be shown to be so in the present example, where the incidence of MI in non-smokers aged 45–49 is at least four times that in non-smokers who are 25–39 years old.[11]

An exception to the general tendency of a greater relative increase in risk at lower levels of baseline risk was the finding that the relative increase associated with heavy smoking in current oral contraceptive users was greater than that among women who never used oral contraceptives or who used them only in the past. This has been noted previously, in that it has been shown that smoking tends to augment the effect of current oral contraceptive use on the risk of MI.[4,12] There was also a suggestion in the data that the effect of heavy smoking may be greater among women with raised total plasma cholesterol levels than among women with lower levels.

Because MI occurs uncommonly in younger women,[11] the public health impact of the increase in incidence due to smoking is limited. For the individual woman, however, the increase in risk incurred by smoking heavily is appreciable, particularly if she is already predisposed to the disease because of other factors.

SUMMARY

The modifying influence of individual risk factors on the relation between myocardial infarction (MI) and cigarette smoking was evaluated in a case-control study of women under 50 years of age: 554 women who had survived first MIs were compared with 2005 hospital controls of similar ages. The risk of MI increased with the number of cigarettes smoked, regardless of the underlying predisposition to MI; the association was apparent at all ages, and in women predisposed to an infarction because of current oral contraceptive use, raised total plasma cholesterol level, decreased high-density lipoproteins, hypertension, diabetes mellitus, blood group A, tendency to type A behaviour, family history of MI, and other factors.

There was clear evidence that current oral contraceptive use substantially augmented the increased risk for smokers. Hypercholesterolaemia may have had the same effect.

ACKNOWLEDGMENTS

This work was supported in part by contract N01-HD-6-2849 with the National Institute of Child Health and Human Development, contract 223-76-3016 with the Food and Drug Administration, and grants-in-aid from Hoffmann-La Roche, Inc, Nutley, NJ, and the Upjohn Company, Kalamazoo, MI.

Nurses, staff, and physicians in 155 hospitals located in the northeastern United States helped with this study. Jacquelyn Smith, MS, coordinated the programme. Marguerite Angeloni, RN, Linda Fields, BSN, Theresa Anderson, RN, Virginia Vida, MEd, and Leonard Gaetano, BChE, assisted with this study.

REFERENCES

[1] Mann JI, Doll R, Thorogood M, Vessey MP, Waters WE. Risk factors for myocardial infarction in young women. Br J Prev Soc Med 1976; 30: 94–100.

[2] Slone D, Shapiro S, Rosenberg L et al. Relation of cigarette smoking to myocardial infarction in young women. N Engl J Med 1978; 298: 1273–6.

[3] Rosenberg L, Shapiro S, Kaufman DW, Slone D, Miettinen OS, Stolley PD. Cigarette smoking in relation to the risk of myocardial infarction in young women. Modifying influence of age and predisposing factors. Int J Epidemiol 1980; 9: 57–63.

[4] Slone D, Shapiro S, Kaufman DW, Rosenberg L, Miettinen OS, Stolley PD. Risk of myocardial infarction in relation to current and discontinued use of oral contraceptives. N Engl J Med 1981; 305: 420–4.

[5] Rosenberg L, Miller DR, Kaufman DW et al. Myocardial infarction in women under 50 years of age. JAMA 1983; 250: 2801–6.

[6] Ischaemic Heart Disease Registers. Report of the Fifth Working Group. Copenhagen: World Health Organization, 1971.

[7] Mantel N, Haenszel W. Statistical aspects of the analysis of data from retrospective studies of disease. J Nat Cancer Inst 1959; 22: 719–48.

[8] Miettinen O. Estimability and estimation in case-referent studies. Am J Epidemiol 1976; 103: 226–35.

[9] Doll R, Peto R. Mortality in relation to smoking: 20 years' observations on male British doctors. Br Med J 1976; 2: 1525–36.

[10] The Pooling Project Research Group. Relationship of blood pressure, serum cholesterol, smoking habit, relative weight and ECG abnormalities to incidence of major coronary events: Final report of the Pooling Project. J Chronic Dis 1978; 31: 201–306.

[11] U.S. Department of Health and Human Services. Vital Statistics of the United States 1977. Vol 2. Mortality. Part A. Hyattsville, Maryland: National Center for Health Statistics, 1981.

[12] Mann JI, Vessey MP, Thorogood M, Doll R. Myocardial infarction in young women with special reference to oral contraceptive practice. Br Med J 1975; 2: 241–5.

Discussion on chapter 12

Vedin

It is quite clear from your presentation that the prevalence of heavy smoking is much more marked in the United States population than in any European population that I know of.

Oliver

I have two questions. One is that lower baseline risk, as measured by a whole variety of characteristics, actually seems to be inversely related to the risk of cigarette smoking. For example, for low HDL the increment with cigarette smoking is appreciably less than it is with high HDL. The other question is, is it true that cigarette smoking is related to infarction and not to angina?

Rosenberg

In response to your first question, among women at lower baseline risk, in general the relative increase seems to be greater. It makes sense to me that if we are talking about an incidence of 5 per 100 000 per year, smoking could increase this tenfold. If you are talking about older people, people aged 70 or more, the relative risk for smoking is about 1.5. Their baseline risk may be perhaps 400 per 100 000 per year, so increasing the risk 50% would increase the incidence to 600 per 100 000 per year. It makes sense to me that when the baseline risk is very low, the relative increase in risk can be very great. The absolute increase is usually greater at higher levels of baseline risk.

In regard to angina, we have not studied it ourselves. It is hard to define angina, as we all know, so it is difficult to study angina in a case-control study. As far as I know though, smoking is not related to angina in the same way as it is to myocardial infarction.

Wilhelmsson

Smoking is a strong risk factor for myocardial infarction in Göteborg, but not at all for angina pectoris, and this applies both to cross-sectional and prospective analyses.

I agree that the diagnosis of angina pectoris is softer than the myocardial infarction diagnosis. We have, however, standardised as much as we can. I would also like to comment on thrombosis in myocardial infarction. Coagulation factors were analysed in 1967 in our prospective population study of men born in 1913. It comes out that fibrinogen is a risk factor in univariate analysis both for stroke and myocardial infarction, but not significant in multivariate analysis when we take smoking, cholesterol levels and blood pressure into account. Fibrinogen is strongly related to smoking and also to cholesterol and blood pressure. Fibrinogen was also a significant risk factor for stroke in multivariate analysis.

Born

Other evidence supports that. T.W. Meade is also finding a strong correlation with fibrinogen within its physiological range.

Rifkind

You mentioned that your analysis assumes no interactions, but in fact cigarette smoking is inversely correlated with HDL levels. Could you comment on how that would affect your relative risk calculations?

Rosenberg

We did not take that into account. We simply looked within levels of HDL to see the effect of smoking. I am not sure that HDL was strongly correlated with smoking in our data.

Rifkind

As I understood the description of the study, the HDL measurements were done in a selected number of subjects some time after hospital discharge. How were the subjects selected? You said you evaluated only some fraction of the anginal subjects. Were these just those people who agreed to participate or was there a sampling scheme? Finally, how did you take into account any alterations in behaviour such as smoking and diet change post infarction?

Rosenberg

We conducted the home interviews at which we obtained blood samples at least 3 months after the infarction, because we had been advised that cholesterol levels would have returned to baseline by that time. Women were selected entirely on the basis of where they lived. We identified certain geographic areas that were safe for our interviewers to go into and eliminated any areas that were not safe or were not convenient, and we ended up thereby including about half of the cases. For each case we selected randomly at least three controls from the same areas as the cases. I think about 80% of eligible cases agreed to participate in this phase and perhaps 70% of the controls.

The smoking data I have presented to you were for smoking habits at the time of hospitalisation—that is, smoking before the myocardial infarction, not after. As to changes in diet, we did ask the women in the home interview if they had changed their diets and a very tiny proportion had. So, if we excluded those women, the results would be unchanged.

Haynes

Have you conducted multivariate analysis on these data? It seems that there are a number of significant interactions, one is a smoking and plasma cholesterol interaction. The relative risks you presented suggest that you may have an atherosclerotic process going on among women rather than a thrombotic process. The relative risk for smokers (more than 25 cigarettes per day) were 11 and 10 for cholesterol levels above 5.2 mmol/l which suggests that the risk is greatest at higher levels of cholesterol. Does smoking work in the absence of high levels of cholesterol?

Rosenberg

Yes, we did do multivariate analysis to control the confounding effects of these multiple risk factors. We did not use it to look at interactions, mainly because we have a hard time understanding what interaction terms mean in multivariate models. They do not have any kind of intuitive meaning to us at the Drug Epidemiology Unit. What we tend to do is look within strata of risk factors, because this has much more meaning for us.

As to why there might be an interaction between smoking and high cholesterol levels, I was hoping that there might be someone in this room who could suggest an explanation.

One of the earliest papers that came out of this study was on women who had no known predisposing conditions. They did not have elevated cholesterol levels, they did not have hypertension, they did not have diabetes, and so on. Among those women, the risks associated with smoking are even greater than the ones that you have seen today. So smoking operates in the complete absence of other risk factors.

Vedin
We are not really surprised, given the inverse relationship between smoking and some other standard risk factors—for instance, the HDL—since it may reflect the selection of infarction patients out of the entire population. Indeed, if you speculate further it might support a causal relationship between tobacco smoking and acute coronary disease in man.

13. Stopping smoking after myocardial infarction in women

C. Wilhelmsson, S. Johansson and A. Vedin

Smoking is a quantitative risk factor for coronary heart disease (CHD), dose-dependent, and synergistic with other major risk factors particularly in young men and women.[1-9] The risk of CHD in people who had stopped smoking was found to decline continuously after discontinuation of smoking.[6,7] Stopping smoking reduces, over time, the increased risk attributable to smoking towards the level of risk in non-smokers. The risk of dying from CHD decreases rapidly after stopping smoking, whereas the risk of dying from lung cancer decreases more slowly.[7] While most of these data relate to men there are sufficient data to provide a basis for a similar conclusion regarding women.

Most younger and middle-aged infarction patients of both sexes are smokers (Table 13.1). In a case-control study of 55 women aged under 50 who had suffered myocardial infarction (MI) the proportion of smokers was 89%, compared with 53% in the controls.

Table 13.1 Numbers of men and women aged under 60 with first myocardial infarction discharged from hospital 1968-77 in relation to preinfarction smoking habits.

Age (years)	Non-smokers		Ex-smokers		Smokers	
	Men	Women	Men	Women	Men	Women
–44	8	6	5	0	109	14
45–49	13	4	13	3	170	21
50–54	37	16	33	8	303	46
55–59	45	22	53	10	320	59
Total	103 (9%)	48 (23%)	104 (9%)	21 (10%)	902 (81%)	140 (67%)

The role of cigarette smoking as a secondary risk factor has been studied extensively in man during the past decade.[10-17] All these studies have shown the beneficial effect of stopping smoking after MI (Table 13.2). A strictly controlled trial of the effects of stopping smoking after MI would ideally require randomisation. Nevertheless, such a study would be very difficult since the large proportion of those advised to stop smoking would not do so while some of those in the control group would probably stop smoking spontaneously. Our initial observations in men[11] have been verified in a larger group of patients with a long follow-up period (Fig. 13.1). There has been no published trial in which the mortality after MI has not been lower in ex-smokers than in continuing smokers. A contrasting finding has been presented by Rose and Hamilton[18] in a randomised trial of primary prevention in civil servants. Stopping smoking was not associated with a reduction in mortality.

Table 13.2 Summary of studies of mortality reduction after myocardial infarction and stopping smoking.

Author	Year	n	Follow-up (years)	Reduction in mortality (%)
Mulcahy et al[10]	1975	252*	4	–
Wilhelmsson et al[11]	1975	405	2	50
Mulcahy et al[12]	1977	190	5	50
Sparrow, Dawber[13]	1978	202	6	60
Pohjola et al[14]	1979	648	5	60
Salonen[15]	1980	523	3	40
Aberg et al[16]	1983	983	10	38
Daly et al[17]	1983	374*	13	55

* Patients with unstable angina are also included

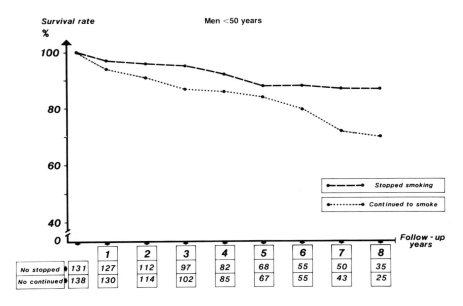

Fig. 13.1 Survival curves for men aged under 50 in relation to smoking status at 3 months after myocardial infarction.

Far less is known about the effects of stopping smoking on mortality and morbidity in women after MI. Sparrow and Dawber[13] reported a 62% reduction in mortality after stopping smoking. The reduction was similar in both men and women. A report from the Helsinki Coronary Register presents a similar reduction in mortality for both sexes after stopping smoking.[14]

GÖTEBORG STUDY

Of 262 women with a first MI discharged alive from hospital in Göteborg between

1968–77, 161 (62%) were smokers at the time of infarction. Post-infarction smoking was confirmed after 3 months. In relation to smoking status 3 months after infarction the subsequent survival and reinfarction rate was calculated by comparing those who smoked before infarction and later stopped (52%) with those who continued to smoke after infarction (48%).

There were no differences in preinfarction characteristics between those who stopped smoking and those who continued. Women who stopped smoking after infarction had higher serum enzyme values during the acute phase than those who continued to smoke.

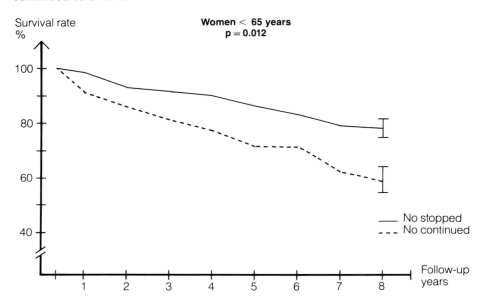

Fig. 13.2 Survival curves for women aged under 65 in relation to smoking status at 3 months after myocardial infarction.

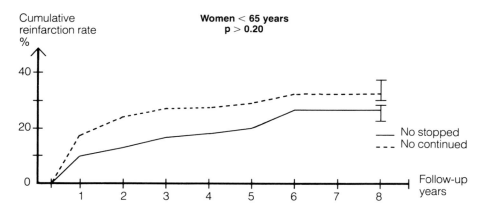

Fig. 13.3 Cumulative reinfarction rates for women aged under 65 in relation to smoking status 3 months after myocardial infarction.

162

The cumulative 8 year survival rate was significantly better in those who stopped compared with those who continued to smoke (p< 0.05, Fig. 13.2). No significant difference was found in the cumulative reinfarction rate between the two groups with different smoking habits (Fig. 13.3).

Conclusion

The beneficial effect of stopping smoking was the same as for men. The effect was seen within a short time period after MI. The differences regarding variables selected to reflect the severity of infarction showed the same pattern as for men. The finding of higher enzyme levels in the group who stopped smoking indicated a more severe than expected prognosis for the group who continued to smoke.

Our findings emphasise the importance of helping patients to stop smoking after MI. Anti-smoking advice is an essential part of patient management. Patients who have not stopped smoking should continuously be informed gently of the increased risk of death. It is important to start anti-smoking information as soon as possible during the hospital stay. All hospital staff should be consistent in the information and advice they give to patients who smoke. Our own positive results have been obtained by giving repeated information both during the hospital stay and in the outpatient clinic. Stopping smoking should be recommended and instituted in all smokers after MI. Women seem to gain at least as much benefit as men from this preventive measure.

REFERENCES

[1]Hammond EC, Horn D. Smoking and death rates—report on forty-four months of follow-up on 187 783 men. I. Total mortality. JAMA 1958; 166: 1159–72.
[2]Doll R, Hill AB. Mortality in relation to smoking: ten years' observations of British doctors. Br Med J 1964; 1: 1460–7.
[3]Doyle JT, Dawber TR, Kannel WB, Kinch SH, Kahn HA. The relationship of cigarette smoking to coronary heart disease. The second report of the combined experience of the Albany, NY, and Framingham, Mass studies. JAMA 1964; 190: 886–90.
[4]Best EWR. A Canadian study of smoking and health. Ottawa Department of National Health and Welfare. 1966: 133.
[5]Kahn HA. The Dorn study of smoking and mortality among U.S. veterans: report on eight and one-half years of observation. In: Haenszel W, ed. Epidemiological approaches to the study of cancer and other chronic diseases. Bethesda, Maryland: National Cancer Institute, 1966; Monograph No 19: 1–126.
[6]Kannel WB, Castelli WP, McNamara PM. Cigarette smoking and risk of coronary heart disease. Epidemiologic clues to pathogenesis. The Framingham Study. In: Wynder EL, Hoffman D, eds. Toward a less harmful cigarette. Bethesda, Maryland: National Cancer Institute, 1968; Monograph No 28: 9–20.
[7]Hammond EC, Garfinkel L. Coronary heart disease, stroke, and aortic aneurysm. Factors in the etiology. Arch Environ Health (Chicago) 1969; 19: 167–82.
[8]Weir JM, Dunn JE Jr. Smoking and mortality: a prospective study. Cancer 1970; 25: 105–12.
[9]Elmfeldt D, Wilhelmsson C, Vedin A, Tibblin G, Wilhelmsen L. Characteristics of representative male survivors of myocardial infarction compared with representative population samples. Acta Med Scand 1976; 199: 387–98.
[10]Mulcahy R, Hickey N, Graham I, McKenzie G. Factors influencing long-term prognosis in male patients surviving a first coronary attack. Br Heart J 1975; 37: 158–65.
[11]Wilhelmsson C, Vedin JA, Elmfeldt D, Tibblin G, Wilhelmsen L. Smoking and myocardial infarction. Lancet 1975; 1: 415–19.
[12]Mulcahy R, Hickey N, Graham IM, MacAirt J. Factors affecting the 5 year survival rate of men following acute coronary heart disease. Am Heart J 1977; 93: 556–9.

[13]Sparrow D, Dawber TR. The influence of cigarette smoking on prognosis after a first myocardial infarction. A report from the Framingham study. J Chronic Dis 1978; 31: 425–32.

[14]Pohjola S, Siltanen P, Romo M et al. Effect of quitting smoking on the long-term survival after myocardial infarction. Trans Eur Soc Cardiol 1979; 1: 2. (Abstract 33)

[15]Salonen JT. Stopping smoking and long-term mortality after acute myocardial infarction. Br Heart J 1980; 43: 463–9.

[16]Aberg A, Bergstrand R, Johansson S et al. Cessation of smoking after myocardial infarction. Effects on mortality after 10 years. Br Heart J 1983; 49: 416–22.

[17]Daly LE, Mulcahy R, Graham IM, Hickey N. Long term effect on mortality of stopping smoking after unstable angina and myocardial infarction. Br Med J 1983; 287: 324–6.

[18]Rose G, Hamilton PJ. A randomised controlled trial of the effect on middle-aged men of advice to stop smoking. J Epidemiol Community Health 1978; 32: 275–81.

Discussion on Chapter 13

de Faire
Were there any differences with regard to personality factors, behaviour pattern or things like that; have you measured that? Alcohol consumption, social factors?

Wilhelmsson
Not in this small female population. In a subset of our male myocardial infarction patients, there was no personality influence. Another interesting finding in our male population is that the patients who continue to smoke have a significantly increased rate of sudden death.

Rifkind
You indicated that there were baseline differences between smokers and non-smokers. To what extent did you explore the potential influence on the prognosis of these baseline differences?

Wilhelmsson
I did show a slide indicating that those who stopped smoking actually had larger infarcts and therefore you would expect a poorer prognosis among them.

Oliver
I just want to be reminded—and you will know the details of Geoffrey Rose's observations in 1979—about the adverse effect in men of stopping smoking. I think he reported that there were more arrhythmic deaths in those who stopped smoking.

Wilhelmsson
Yes, but this population had stopped smoking after myocardial infarction, so you cannot compare it.

14. Sex differences in atherosclerosis

N.H. Sternby

In spite of the predominance of atherosclerotic cardiovascular disease among men it is not in all arteries that men have more extensive and severe atherosclerosis than women. This holds particularly for the aorta, but there are even studies that show coronary atherosclerosis predominates in women. It may therefore be of interest to review the differences between the sexes in atherosclerosis of the various arteries.

This report is based on results of three studies: 'Geographic pathology of atheroslerosis' (McGill 1968),[1] 'Atherosclerosis in a defined population, an autopsy survey in Malmö, Sweden' (Sternby 1968),[2] and 'Atherosclerosis of the aorta and coronary arteries in five towns' (Kagan et al, 1976).[3]

When taking both qualitative and quantitative measurements into account it is well known that atherosclerosis increases with age. Up to age 20 only a few atherosclerotic lesions are present but in the third decade there is a rapid development in both men and women but with men predominating, at least in Western-type populations.

Sex differences in aortic atherosclerosis estimated in this way are found mainly between the ages of 40–69. More information is obtained, however, if the extent of the different types of lesions is estimated. In the aorta the dominating lesion in a Western population up to age 40 is the lipid streak, but thereafter the fibrous plaque. Complicated and calcified lesions appear regularly in men in the 5th and in women in the 6th decade. There are practically no sex differences in the extent of the lipid streaks and fibrous plaques but complicated lesions in almost all age groups are more extensive in men than in women. Calcified lesions are, however, more

Table 14.1 Significant sex differences (males > females) in extent of atherosclerotic lesions of abdominal aorta.

		Type of lesion			
Age (years)	Total extent	Lipid streaks	Fibrous plaques	Compl. lesions	Calc. lesions
30–39					
40–49				*	
50–59				**	
60–69				***	[*]
70–79	[*]			***	***
80–89	[***]	**		*	[***]

[ ] denotes females > males.

extensive in elderly women than in men (Table 14.1). As far as the so-called raised lesions are concerned—that is, all types except the fatty streaks—European men generally have more than European women (Table 14.2) but Malmö is an exception. Of the 19 populations in the International Atherosclerosis Project[1] six showed more aortic involvement of raised lesions among men than women, nine populations showed the opposite, and in four there were practically no differences. It seems that the male preponderance is more pronounced in populations with a high incidence of atherosclerosis than in populations where the general level of atherosclerosis is low.

Table 14.2 Intertown comparisons of the extent of raised lesions (% of surface) in the average aorta and average coronary artery and prevalence (%) of stenosis in any coronary artery in high and low atherosclerosis groups (age-standardised values).

Town	Extent of raised lesions in average aorta		Extent of raised lesions in average coronary artery		Prevalence of stenosis in any coronary artery	
	High group	Low group	High group	Low group	High group	Low group
	Men					
Malmö	44	24	53	24	72	7
Prague	47	32	62	26	57	9
Ryazan	37	26	54	26	53	7
Yalta	37	27	48	23	51	11
Tallin	44	30	52	31	44	10
	Women					
Malmö	49	29	39	15	41	6
Prague	40	24	37	20	26	5
Ryazan	33	15	32	11	13	2
Yalta	34	21	37	12	45	8
Tallin	41	27	42	20	18	9

The role of the fatty streak in the development of aortic atherosclerosis has been much debated over the years. This problem was also studied in the International Atherosclerosis Project.[1] In all populations fatty streaks were more extensive in women than in men, even in those populations where raised lesions were significantly more extensive in men in older age groups. There is still controversy about the possible development of these fatty lesions into more advanced lesions.

On the whole, results of different studies of coronary atherosclerosis are easier to interpret: almost all show that men have more atherosclerosis of the coronary arteries than women (Table 14.2). The sex difference is statistically significant in more age groups than for the aorta, and in the left anterior descending coronary artery as early as the 4th decade (Table 14.3). The extent of the various types of lesions shows that the fibrous plaque is the dominating lesion both in men and women and the pattern of sex differences for the individual lesions is very different from that of the aorta: all lesions except the lipid streaks are significantly more extensive in men, even the fibrous plaque and the calcified lesion (Table 14.4). The prevalence of coronary stenosis is also much higher in men than in women (Table 14.2). The International Atherosclerosis Project[1] also showed that men had much more extensive raised lesions in the coronary arteries than women. The only

Table 14.3 Significant sex differences (males > females) in degree of atherosclerosis of coronary arteries.

Age (years)	Combined arteries	LAD	LC	RC
30–39		*		
40–49	**	**	**	**
50–59	**	**	**	**
60–69	**	**	**	**
70–79	*	**	*	
80–89				

LAD=left anterior descending coronary artery
LC=left circumflex coronary artery
RC=right coronary artery

exception is in the Sao Paulo negro population and there were a couple of other populations where the differences were rather small. In the white North-American population, on the other hand, there was a more than twofold difference. Again, it seemed as if the sex difference grew bigger if the general level of atherosclerosis in a population was increased.

Table 14.4 Significant sex differences (males >females) in extent of atherosclerotic lesions of coronary arteries

Age (years)	Total extent			Lipid streaks			Fibrous plaques			Compl. lesions			Calc. lesions		
	LAD	LC	RC	LAD	LC	RC	LAD	LC	RC	LAD	LC	RC	LAD	LC	RC
20–29				[**]											
30–39	*						*								
40–49	***	***	***	*	*		***	***	***	**	*				
50–59	***	***	***				***	***	***	**	*	**	**	**	**
60–69	***	**	***	[**]		[*]	**	*	***	**	*		***	*	**
70–79					[*]	[***]				**	*		***	*	
80–89			[*]		[*]	[*]									

LAD=left anterior descending coronary artery .
LC=left circumflex coronary artery
RC=right coronary artery
[ ]denotes females>males

The fatty streak in the coronary arteries has also been studied in detail and again the pattern is not absolutely clear. In some populations men have more extensive fatty lesions than women but in most populations women have more and sometimes much more. It seems, however, that in populations with a high degree of coronary heart disease the fatty streak is more likely to develop into fibrous plaques than in other populations but this problem needs further study.

The pattern of the development of cerebral atherosclerosis with increasing age is the same as in other arteries but the rate of increase is slower and there is practically no sex difference even though the prevalence of lipid streaks and fibrous plaques is somewhat higher in men than in women up to age 65 or so.

The peripheral arteries, that is, the carotid and renal arteries and the pelvic and leg arteries, follow the same pattern of development as other arteries and regarding sex differences the pattern is more similar to that of the coronary arteries than to the aorta. There are therefore significant sex differences in ages between 40–70 and sometimes even in the older age groups.

When interpreting the results of these studies one must be aware of two things. The first is that they are based on group observations and however homogeneous a group one tries to select, there is a large individual variation in the extent and severity of atherosclerosis. Part of this variation may reflect the genetic constitution. It is also important to realise that the extent and type of lesions varies with the cause of death. In an epidemiological study control of this factor is therefore important.

The second is that the results are based only on macroscopical examination of the arteries. Much more information is obtained when microscopy and a variety of specialised methods are applied. Such studies are, of course, much more time-consuming and difficult to organise but they are now under way on an international level[4] using a whole battery of sophisticated methods which will be applied to autopsy material from different parts of the world.

REFERENCES

[1]McGill HC Jr. The geographic pathology of atherosclerosis. Baltimore: Williams & Wilkins, 1968.
[2]Sternby NH. Atherosclerosis in a defined population. An autopsy survey in Malmö, Sweden. Acta Pathol Microbiol Immunol Scand 1968; suppl 194: 7–216.
[3]Kagan AR, Sternby NH, Uemura K, Vanécék R, Vihert AM. Atherosclerosis of the aorta and coronary arteries in five towns. Bull WHO 1976; 53: 485–645.
[4]Sternby NH. Protocol for the WHO/ISFC study of the pathobiological determinants of atherosclerosis in youth.

Discussion on Chapter 14

Born

That is enormously interesting. Could it be that a male/female difference is ultimately in the constitution of the lesion, so that the male lesion has elements in it which makes it more liable to disaster?

Sternby

We don't know yet. There are no good studies showing this, they are under way. These results are based mainly on macroscopical grading and what macroscopically looks like similar fibrous lesions may in fact be very different lesions from the point of view of microscopy and biology.

Born

We are engaged in planning a study to look at the difference in constitution in relation to what happens to the lesions, but perhaps one has to subdivide it into males and females.

Sternby

Yes, most studies have not done that. Maybe there is a difference.

Rifkind

Is there a potential problem in these types of data which are obviously derived from people who have died. Could you comment on the extent to which you feel that these data could be compromised by the fact that the younger subjects might be expected to have died from road accidents or trauma deaths in which alcohol would be frequent, that the middle-aged subjects presumably overrepresent myocardial infarction, and that malignancy is more frequent in the older subjects.

Sternby

These studies tried to identify groups of causes of death, because there is a definite difference in the extent of atherosclerosis if you die from coronary heart disease or other atherosclerosis-related diseases or from accidents, cancer etc. These studies have tried to create a basal group mainly consisting of deaths from accidents, cancer and some infectious diseases, to represent the baseline of atherosclerosis in a population. I admit that even in doing this there is a tremendous individual variation which can never be avoided. You may remember that in the 1940s and 1950s a lot of discussion took place whether or not there was a biological inverse relationship between atherosclerosis and cancer? Patients dying from a wasting cancer have less atherosclerosis than others, but I think they constitute a kind of basal level of atherosclerosis and that those who die from myocardial infarction have an increased amount. In the future we will concentrate on accidental deaths to get as clean basal data as possible.

Rifkind

Have you taken into account the various social and economic biases relating to accidental death?

Sternby
We will try to get this information in our future studies.

Vedin
The only way is to work in an environment where the autopsy rate generally is high.

Epstein
There is a great deal of concern now to see what will happen in the next 10 years to the trend of coronary heart disease in men and women in different countries. There are now quite good non-invasive methods to measure changes in atherosclerosis in peripheral vessels.

To what extent can one measure changes over time in the incidence of coronary disease by monitoring changes in the carotid and peripheral vessels by means of non-invasive methods? The crucial question is to what extent these changes mirror what goes on in the coronary arteries. What correlation is there in both men and women between the extent of lesions at one point in time and over time between the coronary and peripheral arteries?

Sternby
The total material shows a good correlation. In the individual patient, however, this does not exist because we know that about 20% of the patients have what I call an irregular distribution of atherosclerosis, that is, they have much in one or two arterial areas but very little in another area. It seems that diabetics and hypertensives are more prone to have an irregular distribution of atherosclerosis.

Epstein
You said something important. If you want to know what happens in the population it does not bother you too much if individual correlations are low.

Sternby
That's right.

Nikkilä
You had included countries with a very low rate of clinical coronary heart disease and countries which have a rather high rate. Have you looked on the nature of the lesions in these two extremes and compared them so that you could say that they are qualitatively similar or different. Could it be a different type of disease in these two extreme cases?

Sternby
It has been done and there are differences. For instance, populations with a high level of atherosclerosis in general have much more of the atheromatous lesion—those with central necrosis. If the intimal surface is not broken they are by definition judged as fibrous lesions but they are more severe, so to speak.

Haynes
I wonder if you could comment on the slide that seemed to suggest that women in

South American countries appear to have a greater degree of fatty streaks than men?

Sternby
Yes, that is true. They have and there is no real explanation for that, nor is there for the black women in the United States who have extensive lipid streaks. But obviously they are not converted into advanced lesions later. We have no explanation for that.

15. Angiographic findings after myocardial infarction in women aged ≤50 years—role of oral contraceptives

H.J. Engel, E. Engel and P.R. Lichtlen

Coronary artery disease in premenopausal women presents two special aspects: the role of oral contraceptives and the problem of normal coronary arteries after unequivocal myocardial infarction (MI).

From several epidemiological studies it has become clear that oral contraceptives significantly increase the risk of cardiovascular morbidity and mortality.[1-5] Some reports have suggested that the risk of MI under oral contraceptive medication concerns primarily those women who have one or more of the commonly acknowledged atherogenic risk factors and who therefore are prone to ischaemic heart disease.[6,7] This might be mediated by the adverse effects of oral contraceptives on blood pressure,[8] and on carbohydrate and lipid metabolism.[9,10] If these side effects of oral contraceptives were responsible for the increased incidence of MI, then it would appear feasible to identify women at risk by an analysis of predisposing atherogenic factors.

The problem of MI while taking oral contraceptives is confounded by angiographic and autoptic observations[11-22] showing the absence of typical atherosclerotic coronary pathology in several of these cases. Thus a differentiation of presence and absence of coronary atherosclerotic changes appears warranted in the analysis of patients who sustained acute MI under oral contraceptive medication.

In an effort to investigate the role of oral contraceptives and of atherogenic risk

Table 15.1 Coronary atherosclerosis (CA) and use of oral contraceptives in the 104 patients of this study.

Cardiac catheterisations
Oct 1974–Oct 1979 (Hanover)
Feb 1981–Mar 1984 (Bremen)
459 women aged ≤ 50 years

Abnormal coronary and/or left ventricular angiograms: n=104

Oral contraceptives		No oral contraceptives	
No CA (n=35)	CA (n=18)	CA (n=42)	No CA (n=9)
Age 38.5 years	Age 42.7 years	Age 45.6 years	Age 41.2 years
Group I	Group II	Group III	Group IV

173

factors with regard to coronary atherosclerosis and MI, we analysed histories, laboratory data and coronary and left ventricular angiograms of 104 women up to the age of 50 years whose angiograms showed unequivocal evidence of coronary atherosclerosis and/or past MI.

In those patients who had sustained MI with normal or almost normal coronary arteries, an attempt was made to answer the question whether abnormalities of the *coagulation system* might be present that made these patients prone to arterial thrombosis. In the same subgroup of patients, we also recorded *24-hour ambulatory ECGs* to find out the incidence of ventricular arrhythmias after MI in the absence of coronary atherosclerosis.

PATIENTS

This report is based on 329 women aged < 50 years who underwent cardiac catheterisation in Hanover Medical University between October 1974 and October 1979[23] and 130 women aged < 50 years who underwent cardiac catheterisation in the division of cardiology of Zentralkrankenhaus 'Links der Weser' in Bremen (FRG) between March 1981 and March 1984. The hospital records of the patients were reviewed and additional correspondence was initiated as necessary to obtain complete clinical information.

Four groups of patients were defined according to oral contraceptive use and the presence or absence of coronary atherosclerosis (Table 15.1):

Group I = MI during oral contraceptive medication; angiographically normal coronary arteries or one isolated focal smooth obstruction of the infarct-related artery, all other brances being entirely normal and free of even minor luminal irregularities (Fig. 15.1).

Group II = MI during oral contraceptive medication; angiographically typical diffuse coronary atherosclerosis with at least 50% obstructions of one or more coronary arteries (Fig. 15.1).

Group III = advanced diffuse coronary atherosclerosis but without (present or past) oral contraceptive medication.

Group IV = MI without (present or past) oral contraceptive medication; angiographically normal coronary arteries or one isolated focal smooth obstruction of the infarct-related vessel, all other branches being entirely normal.

Of the total 459 patients, 35 were allocated to group I (mean age 38.5±4.9 years), 18 to group II (mean age 42.7±5.4 years), 42 group III (mean age 45.6±3.1 years) and 9 to group IV (mean age 41.2±5.0 years). 324 patients had been catheterised because they had valvular or congenital heart disease or because they had normal findings. 31 patients had to be excluded because of incomplete data or previous use of oral contraceptives.

The oral contraceptives used by the patients of groups I and II contained 50 mg ethinyloestradiol with the exception of 1 patient of group II who used a preparation with 100 mg mestranol. The progesterone-only pill was not used by any of the patients.

174

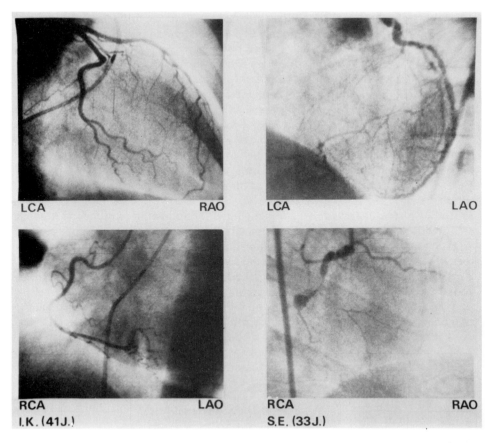

Fig. 15.1 Typical examples of coronary arteriography after myocardial infarction without (left) and with (right) coronary atherosclerosis. LCA=left coronary artery, RCA=right coronary artery, LAO=left anterior oblique projection, RAO=right anterior oblique projection.

METHODS

Clinical observations included the following:

History: family history of premature atherosclerosis (defined as positive if one or both parents and/or siblings had sustained an MI before age 55); gynaecological history including information about the time of first menstruation, pregnancies, menstrual history, history of gynaecological surgery and contraceptive practice; measurement of smoking habit (positive smoking history=more than 10 pack-years); history of chest pain and of MI.

Laboratory tests included an ECG, determinations of serum glucose, glucose chronically above 90 mm Hg, and/or systolic blood pressure chronically above 140 mm Hg.

Laboratory tests included an ECG, determinations of serum glucose, glucose tolerance test and cholesterol (upper limits of normal were taken to be 6.5 mmol/l).

175

Analysis of atherogenic risk factors was confined to the following five parameters: family history, cigarette smoking, hypercholesterolaemia, glucose intolerance and hypertension (all defined as stated above).

Coronary and left ventricular angiography was performed bv the Judkins or Sones techniques, the left ventriculograms (biplane) preceding coronary arteriography. Segmental wall motion was analysed by systolic halfaxial shortening of six halfaxes drawn perpendicularly on the long axis from the mitral-aortic valve junction to the apex at 25, 50 and 75% of its length.[24] Hypokinesis was defined as 10–25% systolic shortening, akinesis as less than 10% shortening. Coronary obstructions were measured with a vernier and refer to percent reduction of luminal diameter.[25] In patients with isolated stenotic lesions, 0.8 mg nitroglycerin (and, after 1978, 10 mg nifedipine as well) was administered in order to exclude coronary spasm.

Studies of the *coagulation system* included the following parameters: number and function of the platelets (thrombometer, platelet aggregation with collagen and ADP, malonyldialdehyde assay, thrombelastogram); plasmatic coagulation factors: thromboplastin test (Quick), partial thromboplastin time (PTT), antithrombin III, plasminogen, fibrinogen, factor VIII:C and factor VIII-associated antigen; and a haemoglobin and haematocrit.

20 of 35 group I patients and 5 of 9 group IV patients participated in the coagulation study which was carried out 9 months to 6 years after MI and discontinuation of oral contraceptive medication.

24-hour ambulatory ECG monitoring was performed in the same 25 patients who volunteered for the coagulation tests. Classification of ventricular arrhythmias was performed according to Lown's criteria[26] modified by Bethge et al:[27]

0 : no ventricular extrasystoles (VES)
I : less than 30 VES/hour
II : more than 30 VES/hour
IIIa : multiform VES
IIIb : bigeminal
IVa : couplets
IVb : salvos
V : R-on-T VES

RESULTS

Group I
MI under oral contraceptive medication but without typical coronary atherosclerosis (n=35).

History
All patients had been on oral contraceptives at the time of their MI. Mean duration of oral contraceptive use was 7.4±4.6 years (6 months to 14 years). Gynaecological history was unremarkable with regard to time of first menstruation and number of pregnancies, deliveries and abortions (only two patients had no children; three patients had had four abortions). There had been no hysterectomies or ovarecto-

mies, and all patients were premenopausal at the time of MI. Only four patients had noted chest pain before MI; 23 patients complained of chest pain which was stress-induced in most cases after MI; surprisingly, post-infarct angina was reported by some patients without any residual haemodynamically significant coronary obstruction.

The number of *atherogenic risk factors* is listed in Table 15.2 and was low with the exception of cigarette smoking.

Table 15.2 Prevalence of atherogenic risk factors.

	Group I (n=35)	Group II (n=42)	Group III (n=9)	Group IV
Cigarette smoking	26	13	34	3
Hypercholesterol-aemia	3	9	20	2
Hypertension	0	12	23	2
Positive family history	8	6	17	0
Glucose intolerance	2	11	23	1

Table 15.3 Coronary anatomy and segmental left ventricular function in groups I–IV. 'Vessels involved' includes normal vessels supplying asynergic left ventricular wall areas in groups I and IV, that is, vessels occluded at the time of myocardial infarction with spontaneously restored vessel patency.

	Group I (n=35)	Group II (n=18)	Group III (n=42)	Group IV (n=9)
Vessels involved	35	40	101	9
MLCA	0	1	3	0
LAD	24	14	41	7
LCx	2	10	25	0
RCA	9	15	32	2
% stenosis				
Normal	10	–	–	3
< 50	9	3	9	1
50–75	3	21	42	3
76–99	7	3	25	2
100	6	13	25	0
Left ventricular function				
Akinesis	23	10	19	6
Hypokinesis	12	8	23	3

MLCA=main left coronary artery
LAD=left anterior descending coronary artery
LCX=left circumflex coronary artery
RCA=right coronary artery

Angiographic findings are summarised in Table 15.3. 29% of the patients had normal coronary arteries, 26% had one isolated luminal irregularity (less than 50% luminal diameter) of the infarct-related vessel. More than 50%, therefore, had no significant coronary obstruction at angiography, which was performed 7 months after MI.

The remaining 55% had isolated smooth focal lesions of more than 50% luminal diameter, the other vessels being normal and free of even minor luminal irregularities. All patients had segmental left ventricular dysfunction corresponding to the ECG location of their MI.

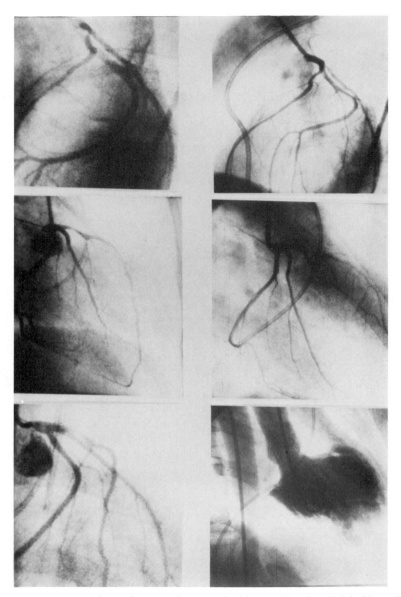

Fig. 15.2 Coronary and left ventricular angiograms of a 36 year-old patient 4 (left side) and 27 (right side) months after myocardial infarction. At the first study (left side: top=LCA LAO, middle and bottom=LCA RAO) there is a 75% proximal LAD stenosis. The second study (right side: top=LCA LAO, middle=LCA RAO, bottom=LV systolic) shows a practically normal LCA and extensive anteroseptal akinesis. Coronary arteriograms at first study after nitroglycerin.

In two cases spontaneous regression of 75% LAD lesions was observed at repeat angiographies performed after intervals of 5 and 23 months. Both patients had experienced extensive anteroseptal infarctions. At repeat angiography both stenoses had regressed to mere luminal irregularities (Figs. 15.2 and 15.3).

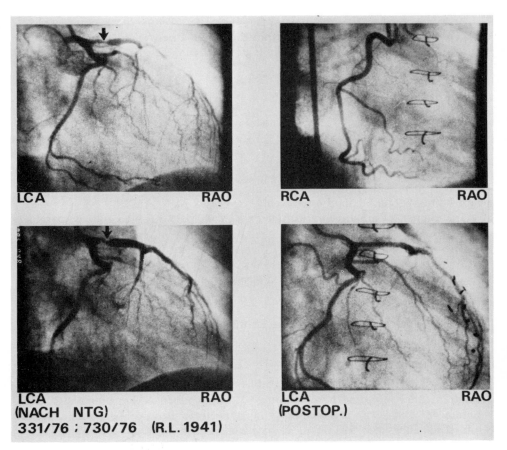

Fig. 15.3 Coronary arteriograms of a 35 year-old woman 7 (left side) and 12 months (right side) after anterior wall myocardial infarction. The patient underwent bypass surgery (to the LAD) and aneurysmectomy between the two studies. The second study shows spontaneous regression of a 75% LAD stenosis. 'NACH NTG'=after nitroglycerin.

Group II

Patients using oral contraceptives with angiographically typical coronary atherosclerosis (n=18).

History

All patients had been on oral contraceptive medication at the time of their MI (mean duration 6.0±2.9 years). All but five had given birth to children. Two patients had undergone hysterectomy, one of them bilateral ovarectomy as well. Two patients were postmenopausal (menopause at age 47 and 48 years). Otherwise gynaecological history was unremarkable. 13 of the 18 patients had complained of angina pectoris before infarction.

The incidence of *atherogenic risk factors* is listed in Table 15.2. In contrast to group I, the prevalence of risk factors was high in group II.

179

Angiographic findings are listed in Table 15.3. There were 37 obstructions greater than 50%, the remaining vessels also showing typical atherosclerotic changes. Four patients had segmental left ventricular dysfunction in the distribution of more than one vessel.

Group III
Advanced diffuse coronary atherosclerosis without oral contraceptive medication (n=42).

History
13 of these patients had no children, four of them had had abortions. Five patients were postmenopausal (menopause at age 41–49). Four patients had undergone hysterectomy, one bilateral ovarectomy.

The number of *atherogenic risk factors* (Table 15.2) was high and comparable with group II.

Angiographic findings (Table 15.3): there were 92 obstructions by more than 50% with typical atherosclerotic changes in the other vessels. More than one region of segmental left ventricular dysfunction was present in six patients.

Group IV
MI without typical coronary atherosclerosis and no history of oral contraceptive medication (n=9).

History
Gynaecological history was unremarkable: all but two patients had given birth to children; there was one hysterectomy, all other patients were premenopausal. Before MI there was premonitory angina pectoris in only one patient. After infarction, chest pain was noted by six patients.

The mean prevalence of *atherogenic risk factors* was as low as in group I (Table 15.2); cigarette smoking was not so predominant.

Angiographic findings (Table 15.3) were also comparable with those of group I.

Coagulation tests
Analysis of platelets regarding number and the various functional tests enumerated above ('methods') did not produce any abnormal findings. The same was true of the thromboplastin test (Quick), antithrombin III, plasminogen, fibrinogen, and factor VIII:C. Partial thromboplastin time (PTT) was shortened ($= 33$ seconds) in nine of the 21 patients (43%) of groups I and IV in whom this test was performed (mean 34.3 ± 2.2 seconds); groups I and IV did not differ in this respect. Factor VIII-associated antigen was increased in eight of 19 patients (42%) (mean $179.5 \pm 100.2\%$,

Table 15.4 Arrhythmias recorded in 20 patients of group I and in 5 patients of group IV.

Lown class:	0	1	II	IIIa	IIIb	IVa	IVb	V
Group I	4	5	0	3	1	4	2	1
Group IV	1	0	0	2	0	1	1	0

normal 50-150%). Factor VIII-associated antigen was abnormal in seven of 16 group I patients and one of three group IV patients.

The results of the *24-hour ambulatory ECG recordings* are summarised on Table 15.4.

DISCUSSION

Among 104 women aged 50 years or younger with angiographically verified MI, 44 (42%) did not have coronary atherosclerosis angiographically (groups I and IV). Coronary arteries were normal in 13 of these cases and there were isolated focal smooth lesions with otherwise completely normal vessels in the other 31 cases. These findings contrast with those of MIs of atherosclerotic aetiology where generalised coronary atherosclerosis of practically all epicardial branches is a universal finding.[28]

Of the 44 patients with MI without coronary atherosclerosis, 35 (80%) had been on oral contraceptives at the time of MI. Of 53 patients who used oral contraceptives at the time of MI 35 (66%) did not have coronary atherosclerosis angiographically. In the latter group, the incidence of atherogenic risk factors—with the exception of cigarette smoking—was low. If the adverse side effects of oral contraceptives on blood pressure[8] and on carbohydrate and lipid metabolism[9,10] had been responsible for these MIs, then it might have been expected that these atherogenic risk factors would be more prevalent in group I patients than they actually were. Data from group I suggest that the analysis of atherogenic risk factors does not produce information about the propensity for cardiovascular side effects of oral contraceptives.

This statement conflicts with the findings of Oliver[6] and Radford and Oliver[7] who report that a high incidence of atherogenic risk factors predisposes to cardiovascular side effects of oral contraceptives; unfortunately, their data lack angiographic confirmation of coronary atherosclerosis.

Comparing groups II and III (coronary atherosclerosis with and without oral contraceptive history), a notable difference in atherogenic risk factors is not apparent. It would be speculative to conjecture about the role of oral contraceptives in group II, but an independent effect in promoting MI cannot be ruled out.

Analysis of the clinical and angiographic data of group I suggests that MI under oral contraceptive medication may be a discrete disease entity unrelated to coronary atherosclerosis. Although oral contraceptives increase the risk of MI, they do not appear to be a typical atherogenic risk factor. In contrast to groups II and III, premonitory angina pectoris was rare in these patients, and the only risk factor present in most patients was cigarette smoking. Synergistic effects of cigarette smoking and oral contraceptives with regard to cardiovascular side effects may be suspected from theoretical considerations and they have been demonstrated in epidemiological studies.[29,30]

Reports of angiographic coronary findings in cases of MI while taking oral contraceptives[16-18,20-22] are comparable with our own observations and show either completely normal vessels or isolated obstructions of otherwise absolutely normal arteries.

Autopsy reports on young women who had been on oral contraceptives at the time of their lethal MI[11-15, 19] universally mention occlusive coronary thrombi, whereas atherosclerotic changes were either absent or only mild. Histology of the coronary vessels was inconsistent with coronary atherosclerosis in these cases. In contrast, autopsy findings after MI of atherosclerotic aetiology demonstrate atherosclerotic changes in practically every segment of the epicardial coronary arteries.[28]

Among the acknowledged side effects of oral contraceptives is a statistically significant increase in venous thrombosis, pulmonary emboli[31] and cerebrovascular accidents[32] by a factor of 8 to 10. It is conceivable that, in rare cases with a hitherto unknown special predisposition, oral contraceptives may also cause thromboembolic coronary occlusions in the absence of coronary atherosclerosis.

The possible mechanisms by which oral contraceptives could produce these events include their effects on serum clotting factors,[33] on the structure of the arterial wall[34] and on platelet adhesiveness.[33]

The observation of spontaneous regression of two 75% proximal LAD lesions is thought to support the hypothesis of thromboembolic occlusions with subsequent thrombolysis as a possible mechanism of myocardial infarction during oral contraceptive medication. A similar case with regression of a 50% LAD stenosis between the 7th and 38th month after an anterior wall infarction was reported by Henderson et al.[20]

An alternative hypothesis for the mechanism of oestrogen-mediated thromboembolism is coronary spasm.[35] Immunological mechanisms have also been accused of being responsible for thrombotic risk related to oral contraceptives.[36]

If the cardiovascular side effects of oral contraceptives are mediated by increased coagulability,[37] recognition of susceptible individuals might be possible by an analysis of the clotting system. Unfortunately, the detailed examination of platelet and plasma factors performed in patients of groups I and IV did not give any promising clues in this respect. The decrease in partial thromboplastin time and the increase in factor VIII-associated antigen[38] observed in some of these patients represent interesting new findings. Even so, they need to be confirmed in a larger number of patients, and interpretation of these data is difficult. The value of the presented studies on coagulation is limited further by the fact that they were performed at variable intervals after discontinuation of oral contraceptives. It would be of more interest to obtain this information during current medication.

Analysis of the gynaecological histories does not offer convincing evidence that ovarian dysfunction may have been a major atherogenic factor in patients of any of the four groups. Premature atherosclerosis was, however, associated with an unusually high incidence of the commonly acknowledged atherogenic risk factors (groups II and III) which confirms earlier observations from the United States.[39] Interestingly, most of these patients had a premonitory history of angina pectoris before their MI which was absent in the patients of groups I and IV.

Ambulatory ECG recordings documented quantitatively and qualitatively abnormal ventricular extrasystoles in 15 of 25 patients (60%) of groups I and IV. Since most of these patients had uncompromised arterial inflow to all regions of myocardium, this indicates that past MIs rather than present ischaemia are responsible for these arrhythmias.

In summary, 42% of young women with MI did not have typical coronary atherosclerosis angiographically; 80% of these patients had been on oral contraceptives at the time of their infarctions.

66% of patients with MI on oral contraceptives did not have coronary atherosclerosis; the incidence of atherogenic risk factors was low in these patients. Hence MI on oral contraceptives appears to be independent of coronary atherosclerosis. The risk of the cardiovascular side effects of oral contraceptives cannot be predicted by an analysis of atherogenic risk factors. This applies also to tests of the coagulation system, although further investigations appear to be warranted.

Although oral contraceptives seem to increase the risk of MI, they are not a typical atherogenic risk factor. Ventricular arrhythmias may persist after MI in spite of the restoration of vessel patency.

Coronary atherosclerosis is rare among premenopausal women; it is associated with an unusually high number of atherogenic risk factors. 30% of the patients had also taken oral contraceptives, but their role remains unclear.

SUMMARY

Coronary arteriography in young women has shown surprisingly frequent cases of myocardial infarction (MI) not associated with coronary atherosclerosis. Among 104 women aged±50 years with a history of acute MI, 60 had coronary atherosclerosis angiographically and 44 did not. According to the coronary anatomy and use of oral contraceptives, the 104 patients were allocated to one of four groups: Groups I and II with contraceptive history without (group I, n=35) and with (group II, n=18) coronary atherosclerosis, groups III and IV without oral contraceptive history with (group III, n=42) and without (group IV, n=9) coronary atherosclerosis. The patients were analysed with regard to their history, the incidence of atherogenic risk factors, and coronary and left ventricular angiograms. In addition, patients of groups I and IV (MI without coronary atherosclerosis) were submitted to an analysis of their coagulation system and of the incidence of ventricular arrhythmias (ambulatory ECG monitoring).

Of 44 patients with MI without coronary atherosclerosis (groups I and IV), 35 had used oral contraceptives at the time of MI; with the exception of cigarette smoking, the incidence of atherogenic risk factors was low in this group. The analysis of atherogenic risk factors and of coagulation tests did not allow an estimation of susceptibility to the cardiovascular side effects of oral contraceptives. The incidence of ventricular arrhythmias was high even with patent vessels.

Young women with typical coronary atherosclerosis (groups II and III) had an unusually high incidence of atherogenic risk factors; oral contraceptives were used by 18 of the 60 patients.

Among patients who had sustained a MI during oral contraceptive medication, 66% did not have coronary atherosclerosis angiographically. Two patients showed spontaneous regression of 75% proximal LAD lesions to mere luminal irregularities after 5 and 23 months. Hence MI while taking oral contraceptives may be a discrete disease entity unrelated to coronary atherosclerosis. Although oral contraceptives appear to increase the risk of MI, they are not a typical atherogenic risk factor.

ACKNOWLEDGMENTS

We thank Dr Barthels and Dr Avenarius of the division of haematology, Hanover Medical University, for performing and evaluating the coagulation tests.

We are indebted to Dr Bethge of the division of cardiology, Göttingen University, who registered and analysed the 24 hour ambulatory ECGs.

REFERENCES

[1] Beral V. Mortality among oral-contraceptive users. Lancet 1977; 2: 727–31.
[2] Vessey MP, McPherson K, Johnson B. Mortality among women participating in the Oxford family planning association contraceptive study. Lancet 1977; 2: 731–3.
[3] Vessey MP, Mann JI. Female sex hormones and thrombosis. Epidemiological aspects. Br Med Bull 1978; 34: 157–62.
[4] Royal College of Practitioners' Oral Contraception Study. Further analyses of mortality in oral contraceptive users. Lancet 1981; 1: 541–6.
[5] Stadel BV. Oral contraceptives and cardiovascular disease. N Engl J Med 1981; 305: 612–8,672–8.
[6] Oliver MF. Oral contraceptives and myocardial infarction. Br Med J 1970; 2: 210–3.
[7] Radford DJ, Oliver MF. Oral contraceptives and myocardial infarction. Br Med J 1973; 3: 428–30.
[8] Saruta T, Saade GA, Kaplan NM. A possible mechanism for hypertension induced by oral contraceptives. Arch Intern Med 1970; 126: 621–6.
[9] Wynn V, Doar JWH. Some effects of oral contraceptives on carbohydrate metabolism. Lancet ·1969; 2: 761–6.
[10] Hennekens CH, Evans DA, Castelli WP, Taylor JO, Rosner B, Kass EH. Oral contraceptive use and fasting triglyceride, plasma cholesterol and HDL cholesterol. Circulation 1979; 60: 486–9.
[11] Hartveit F. Complications of oral contraception. Br Med J 1965; 1: 60–1.
[12] Naysmith JH. Oral contraceptives and coronary thrombosis. Br Med J 1965; 1: 250.
[13] Osborn GR. Oral contraception and thrombosis. Br Med J 65; 1: 1128.
[14] Dalgaard JB, Gregersen M. Coronarthrombose nach hormonaler Antikonzeption. Beitr Gerichtl Med 1967; 25: 224–34.
[15] Stout C. Coronary thrombosis without coronary atherosclerosis. Am J Cardiol 1969; 24: 564–9.
[16] Dear HD, Jones WB. Myocardial infarction associated with the use of oral contraceptives. Ann Intern Med 1971; 74: 236–9.
[17] Glancy DL, Marcus ML, Epstein SE. Myocardial infarction in young women with normal coronary arteriograms. Circulation 1971; 44: 495–502.
[18] Waxler EB, Kimbiris D, van den Broek H, Segal BL, Likoff W. Myocardial infarction and oral contraceptive agents. Am J Cardiol 1971; 28: 96–101.
[19] Weiss S. Myocardial infarction and oral contraceptives. N. Engl J Med 1972; 286; 436–7.
[20] Henderson RR, Hansing CE, Razavi M, Rowe GG. Resolution of an obstructive coronary lesion as demonstrated by selective angiography in a patient with transmural myocardial infarction. Am J Cardiol, 1973; 31: 785–8.
[21] Maleki M, Lange RL. Coronary thrombosis in young women on oral contraceptives: Report of two cases and review of the literature. Am Heart J 1973; 85: 749–54.
[22] Ciraulo DA. Recurrent myocardial infarction and angina in a woman with normal coronary angiograms. Am J Cardiol 1975; 35: 923–6.
[23] Engel H-J, Engel E, Lichtlen PR. Coronary atherosclerosis and myocardial infarction in young women—role of oral contraceptives. Eur Heart J 1983; 4: 1–8.
[24] Herman MV, Heinle RA, Klein MD, Gorlin R. Localized disorders in myocardial contraction. Asynergy and its role in congestive heart failure. N Engl J Med 1967; 277: 222–32.
[25] Rafflenbeul W, Heim R, Dzuiba M, Henkel B, Lichtlen P. Morphometric analysis of coronary arteries. In: Lichtlen PR, ed. Coronary angiography and angina pectoris. Stuttgart: George Thieme, 1976: 255–64.

[26]Lown B, Wolf M. Approaches to sudden death from coronary heart disease. Circulation 1971; 44: 130–42.

[27]Bethge KP, Klein H, Lichtlen PR. Koronare Herzerkrankung, Rhythmusstörungen und plözlicher Herztod. Intern Welt 1979; 2: 107–17.

[28]Roberts WC, Buja LM. The frequency and significance of coronary arterial thrombi and other observations in fatal acute myocardial infarction. Am J Med 1972; 52: 425–43.

[29]Frederiksen H, Ravenholt RT. Thromboembolism, oral contraceptives, and cigarettes. Public Health Rep 1970; 85: 197–206.

[30]Mann JI, Vessey MP, Thorogood M, Doll R. Myocardial infarction in young women with special reference to oral contraceptive practice. Br Med J 1975; 2: 241–5.

[31]Vessey MP, Doll R. Investigation of relation between use of oral contraceptives and thromboembolic disease; a further report. Br Med J 1969; 2: 651–7.

[32]Masi AT, Dugdale M. Cerebrovascular diseases associated with the use of oral contraceptives. Ann Intern Med 1970; 72: 111–21.

[33]Dugdale M, Masi AT. Effects of oral contraceptives, advisory committee on obstetrics and gynecology. Washington, DC: Food and Drug Administration, 1969: 43–51.

[34]Irey NS, Manion WC, Taylor HB. Vascular lesions in women taking oral contraceptives. Arch Pathol 1970; 89: 1–8.

[35]Jaffe MD. Effect of oestrogens on postexercise electrocardiogram. Br Heart J 1977;38: 1299–303.

[36]Beaumont JL, Beaumont V. Immunological mechanisms and CHD in young women. In: Oliver MF, ed. Coronary heart disease in young women. Edinburgh, London, New York: Churchill Livingstone, 1978: 145–50.

[37]Poller L. Oral contraceptives, blood clotting and thrombosis. Br Med Bull 1978; 34: 151–6.

[38]Nilsson IM. Report of the working party on factor VIII— related antigens. Thromb Haemost 1978; 39: 511–20.

[39]Engel HJ, Page HL, Campbell WB. Coronary artery disease in young women. JAMA 1974; 230: 1531–4.

Discussion on chapter 15

Vedin
One question that arises regards the recruitment of patients. Your conclusion requires that you can examine a sizeable proportion of the cases with myocardial infarction on a contraceptive medication. Could you give us a little bit information on how you recruited the patients?

Engel
This is primarily an angiographic observation. I went through the cath-lab data and I picked—that was the cohort—all the catheterised patients since 1974 and I looked at all the patients who were younger than 50 and studied them.

Beaumont J.-L.
Have you any other data on the possible implication of spasm in this disease?

Engel
Well, clinically they did not appear to have the Prinzmetal type of angina. They did not have variant angina in the sense of having episodes of pain unrelated to effort. They had one big event and in only 11% of the patients angina pectoris was present before myocardial infarction. I cannot exclude the possibility that spasm may have played a role, but as far as the history is concerned these patients did not have variant angina.

Shapiro
Did you look at the duration of oral contraceptive use in those patients with infarcts in whom atheroma was present and those in whom it was absent?

Engel
In those in whom atheroma was absent, group I, the mean duration of oral contraceptive medication was 7.2 years, with a range of 6 months to 14 years. In the second group it was 6 years.

Shapiro
Ignoring people presently taking oral contraceptives, it would be interesting to know the duration of past oral contraception.

Engel
I did not have a single patient who had taken oral contraceptives at some time in the past. They were excluded.

Sternby
Have you got any material from similar groups who died from myocardial infarction? It would give you a clue to the presence of thrombus without athero-sclerosis.

Engel
Yes, there are some post mortem reports and they all mention the presence of

thrombotic material and they almost universally mention the absence of typical atherosclerotic lesions.

Wynn

I think it is nice of you to refer to women with an average age of 40 as young women. I am sure that is a good thing. How would your data compare if you studied young men? Is there any difference in this mysterious disease which kills young women, or certainly disables them. They have normal coronary arteries according to your thesis but they are either destroyed or pretty ill by myocardial infarction of mysterious origin. How does it compare with young men?

Engel

It is, I think, a surprise angiographic finding. Many people have seen that the incidence of single-vessel disease, or maybe even normal coronary artery disease, is fairly high in young men as well.

Wynn

How did you diagnose myocardial infarction in your women?

Engel

By history, by enzymes, by ECG, by left ventriculograms, angiographic findings. All were concordant.

Wynn

You had enzymes in every case?

Engel

They were typical. They had unequivocal myocardial infarction.

Wynn

I must refer to something that has been happening at my hospital for three or four years. For years our cardiologists sent back reports on the ECGs on large groups of young women on oral contraceptives. The reports that we were getting back indicated widespread ischaemic changes, anterolateral myocardial infarction—you name it, we have got reports on it. These were usually symptomless and healthy young women. I can remember one patient with chest pain in whom we in fact thought that she had had an episode of myocardial infarction judged by electrocardigraphic changes. She had a normal coronary angiogram. We have now come to the conclusion that the interpretation of the ECG in young women is quite difficult and certainly the exercise ECG may be equally misleading. The ordinary resting ECGs can show a high prevalence of so-called abnormalities which are probably not abnormalities at all in the real sense.

Vedin

One of the answers might be that you should perhaps get another cardiologist.

Wynn

I did. We sent these cardiograms around to five cardiologists and it was only after they got together that they then realised that for years they had been reporting these ECGs in young women as being abnormal.

Engel

Do they refer to ST changes? Do they refer to abnormalities of the QRS complex?

Vedin

That could be most ST segments. Dr Johansson will have some information on female/male angiographic comparisons.

Johansson

We have compared cardioangiographic findings in 50 women and 69 men aged 40–54 years with myocardial infarction. The female patients less often had left ventricular wall motion abnormalities than the male patients. No sex difference was found in the prevalence of coronary artery abnormalities, although women tended to have more normal coronary arteries than men. In this series about 20% of the female patients had completely normal coronary arteries.

Engel

Had they undergone myocardial infarctions?

Johansson

Yes, all patients had suffered a myocardial infarction. Can you explain on what basis patients with proximal LAD stenosis in groups I and IV were grouped together with those of normal coronary arteries? Furthermore, what was the difference in risk factors between patients with LAD stenosis and those with completely normal coronary arteries?

Engel

I did not specifically analyse that point. As I showed in my two examples, there is a transition from a proximal LAD stenosis to completely normal coronary arteries. I think angiographically you could make a clear distinction between typical diffuse coronary atherosclerosis and the isolated focal smooth lesion that these groups of patients had, with otherwise completely normal coronary arteries. That is a clear difference.

de Faire

I think your figure of 42% of the young females with myocardial infarction who did not have the coronary atherosclerosis was surprisingly high. We find about 25% in the Stockholm area. Could this difference be due to the classification in any way? Do you include coronary plaques, for example, in your classification?

Engel

Yes, if they do have more than one plaque then they are group II or III.

Haynes
In the Duke University angiography study we have compared women with absolutely clean arteries with those with 50% stenosis or more. We found that there were no differences between groups on a number of psychological measures including the MMPI hysteria, hyperchondriasis, depression and neuroticism scales as well as type A behaviour scales in older women. We do find a significant correlation in type A behaviour in the diseased group (more type A) among younger women (aged 35–44) and wondered if you had any psychological measures in your data. Did you refer to some social measures? Were the younger women, for example, more likely to be working women or housewives or employed in high occupational jobs rather than low occupational jobs?

Engel
I have no information about that.

Rifkind
I am a bit concerned about describing women as having no risk factors if their cholesterol is below 6.5 mmol/l. I do not have precise data to hand but only the top few percent of 30–39 year-old women would exceed 6.5. Levels above 6 mmol/l or so are high. I do not think that this necessarily alters your findings but the notion that such women are free of all coronary risk factors is not justified.

Engel
You have to have a cutoff point somewhere. 4.7 is better than 5.2. I think 6.5 is the generally accepted point.

Rifkind
An approach where you treated the cholesterol levels continuously rather than dichotomously might be helpful.

16. Oral contraception and thrombosis: implication of anti sex-steroid hormone antibodies

V. Beaumont and J.-L. Beaumont

Oral contraceptive use is associated with an increased risk of thrombosis in all the circulatory system, involving venous as well as arterial vessels.[1-3]

A direct relationship between myocardial infarction (MI) and the pill, suspected as early as 1963,[4] was supported by several case reports[5-9] and soundly confirmed by epidemiological studies.[10-12]

Ischaemic heart disease is known to be associated with several risk factors. The suggestion was made that women who suffered from ischaemic heart disease on the pill were women with factors predisposing to atherosclerosis.

On the other hand, the possibility of an immunological mechanism was suggested in 1976[13] in a patient with pulmonary thrombosis and serum antiethinyloestradiol antibodies. Further studies confirmed the association between such antibodies and the thrombotic events in women on oral contraceptives.[14]

In the present work, the respective role of risk factors of atherosclerosis and anti-steroid hormone antibodies will be compared in women with MI and thrombosis of other organs.

SOURCES OF INFORMATION

Patients

Between 1978 and 1983 the serum from more than a thousand women was referred to our research group from 82 medical departments all over France. These women had been discharged with a diagnosis of thrombosis while on oral contraceptives or other synthetic sex hormones.

For 468 of them the diagnosis was ascertained by clinical, angiographic or electrocardiographic documents. 20 of those 468 patients presented with ischaemic heart disease compared with 220 with cerebrovascular disease, 187 with venous and/or pulmonary embolism, and 41 with systemic venous or arterial thrombosis of other localisation (Table 16.1).

The relative frequency of coronary heart disease cannot be estimated from these data. Women were not recruited on pre-established criteria and our laboratory may have a better response from neurologists than cardiologists.

Table 16.1 Thrombosis in women on synthetic sex hormones (1978-83).

Ischaemic heart disease		20
Cerebrovascular disease		
stroke	151	
transient cerebral ischaemia	35	220
other thrombosis	34	
Venous thromboembolic disease		
with predisposing factors	9	
without predisposing factors		
–venous thrombosis	113	187
–pulmonary thrombosis or embolism	65	
Miscellaneous		
systemic arterial or venous thrombosis	30	41
Budd Chiari syndrome	11	
Total cases		468

It must be noticed, however, that the attributable risk of oral contraceptives estimated by Stadel[15] from several retrospective and prospective studies was 37 per 10 000 women/year for stroke, 49 for venous thrombosis and only seven cases for MI under 39. The risk increased sharply to 67 only after 40 years.

The clinical features of the ischaemic heart disease in the 20 patients is given in Table 16.2.

Table 16.2 Synthetic sex hormones and coronary heart disease, clinical aspects.

	Non-menopausal women Oral contraception	Menopausal women Substitutive treatment	Men
No of cases	13	6	1
Myocardial infarction	10	2	1
Impending infarction	1	3	
Angina pectoris	2	1	

— All women received synthetic sex hormones either for oral contraception (13 women), as a substitutive treatment with synthetic oestrogens and/or progestogens (six non-menstruating women) or other reason (one man of 33 years on heavy oestrogen therapy).

— All of them had confirmed myocardial or impending infarction except three women who presented with angina pectoris (15%). Women on oral contraceptives were, of course, younger (mean age 33.7, ranging from 23–46 years) than women on substitutive treatment (mean age 50.3 ranging from 30–59 years).

Classical risk factors of ischaemic heart disease were looked for: serum cholesterol levels of above 6.5 mmol/l (250 mg/100 ml), hypertension above 160 mm Hg for systolic and 90 for diastolic blood pressure, hyperglycaemia, and cigarette smoking. Besides, the presence of serum antiethinyloestradiol antibodies (anti-EO ab) was investigated by a radioimmunoassay using tritiated ethinyloestradiol.[16]

In cases of MI these factors were compared in women on oral contraceptives and in menopausal women on a substitutive treatment.

191

The group of 13 women with MI while on oral contraceptives was also compared with groups of oral contraceptive users with thrombosis of other localisation for whom full information was obtainable: 19 cases of cerebrovascular thrombosis and 17 cases of venous thrombosis.

RESULTS

Risk factors in patients with coronary heart disease

(Tables 16.3 and 16.4)
The classical risk factors associated with coronary heart disease were not equally distributed among the three groups of women on oral contraceptives, the meno-pausal women treated with synthetic sex hormones, and the man.

High serum cholesterol, high blood pressure and diabetes were essentially found in older women: four women out of six had hypercholesterolaemia, two out of six had hypertension, and two out of six had diabetes; in younger women on oral contraceptives only one had both hypercholesterolaemia and hypertension.

On the other hand, smoking habits were much more frequent in contraceptive users (11 women out of 13) than in older women (one out of six).

Finally, the characteristic common to nearly all patients was the presence of serum antibodies to ethinyloestradiol, which were found in 12 out of 13 women on the pill, five out of the six women on substitutive treatment, and also in the man who had no other risk factors except smoking.

Risk factors in other localisations

The same risk factors were compared in oral contraceptive users with different types of thrombosis.

Only minor and non-significant differences were seen between the groups (Table 16.5): women with arterial coronary or cerebrosvascular thrombosis were older; the duration of oestroprogestative use was shorter in women with venous thrombosis, and cholesterol levels were higher in MI.

The percentage of smokers was higher in women with MI (76.9%) than in the groups with venous (58.8%) or cerebrovascular (52.6%) disease. The mean number of cigarettes per day was also significantly higher in coronary heart disease (14 ± 10) than in thrombophlebitis (6 ± 8) ($p < 0.05$).

The most frequent finding was anti-EO ab present in 92% of coronary cases, 84% of cerebrovascular diseases, and 88% of venous thrombosis.

So, two factors emerged in women with thrombosis on oral contraceptives: cigarette smoking and, especially, anti-EO ab.

IMPLICATIONS OF IMMUNOLOGICAL FACTORS IN THE DEVELOPMENT OF THROMBOSIS

A monoclonal IgG λ with antiethinyloestradiol activity was first shown in 1976 in a 36 year-old woman with pulmonary embolism while on oral contraceptives.[13]

Table 16.3 Coronary heart disease (CHD) in 13 women on oral contraceptives.

Case no	Age (years)	CHD	Oral contraceptives Duration of use* (months)	Dose of oestrogen (µg)	Serum cholesterol (mmol/l)	(mg/100 ml)	Risk factors Blood pressure ≥160 mm Hg	Cig/day	Anti-EO ab (cpm)
1	43	MI	92	50	6.2	240	0	10	995
2	23	MI	4	30	5.1	198	0	0	1130
3	40	MI	84	–	5.7	220	0	7	926
4	28	MI	9	30	6.2	240	0	20	790
5	46	MI	3	30	5.8	225	0	0	2371
6	34	AP	120	50	5.2	200	0	40	654
7	23	MI	3	50	6.0	230	0	5	97
8	35	AP	90	30	6.0	230	+	12	0
9	29	MI	98	50	6.1	235	0	20	548
10	39	II	?	30	6.1	235	0	15	426
11	32	MI	132	50	6.2	240	0	20	488
12	35	MI	264	30	6.3	245	0	20	382
13	32	MI	84	30	5.1	198	0	20	225

MI=myocardial infarction
AP=angina pectoris
II=impending infarction
* Oestroprogestative hormones, except case 3 (progestative pill)

Table 16.4 Coronary heart disease (CHD) in six hormone-treated menopausal women and in a young man on synthetic sex hormones.

Case no	Age (years)	CHD	Treatment Duration (months)	Hormones	Risk factors Serum cholesterol (mmol/l)	(mg/100 ml)	Blood pressure ≥160 mm Hg	Diabetes n cases	Cig/day	Anti-EO ab (cpm)
1	51	II	36	O	8.3	320	0	0	0	289
2	48	II	34	O	6.9	267	0	0	0	872
3	59	II	48	P	5.1	196	0	0	0	495
4	39	MI	72	O	5.1	198	0	+	40	765
5	52	MI	18	P	7.3	280	+	+	0	0
6	53	AP	60	O	11.9	460	+	0	0	447
Man	33	MI	?	O+P	6.2	240	0	0	10	274

MI=myocardial infarction
AP=angina pectoris
II=impending infarction
O=oestrogens
P=progestogens

Table 16.5 Oral contraception (OC) and thrombosis. Risk factors in different localisations.

	n	Age (years)	Duration of OC (months) m±	Serum cholesterol (mmol/l) m±	(mg/100 ml) m±	High BP ≥160 mm Hg n cases	Cig/day m±	Anti-EO ab n positive cases (%)
Cerebrovascular diseases	19	33±8	82±74	53±1.1	205±44	1	10±16	16 (84)
Ischaemic heart disease	13	34±7	76±60	5.8±0.4	236±33	1	14±10	12 (92)
Venous thrombosis and/or pulmonary embolism	17	28±7	61±39	5.5±0.7	213±27	0	6±8	15 (88)

*p<0.05

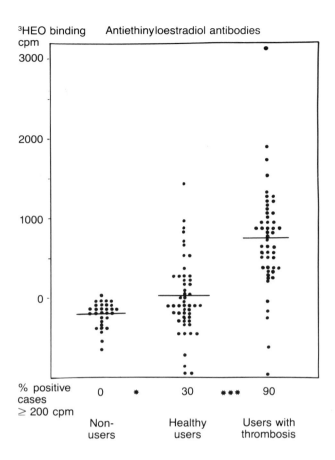

Fig. 16.1 Binding of tritiated ethinyloestradiol (3HEO) in oral contraceptive users and non-users. *p < 0.05, *** p < 0.001.

From this time further studies were conducted to evaluate the frequency of the antibodies in the population of oral contraceptive users. A simple detection of circulating immune complexes (CIC) by serum precipitation in ammonium sulphate at 25% saturation showed that in oral contraceptive users about 25% were immunoreactive, compared with 90% in women with thrombosis.[17,18] This simple but unspecific method was later changed for a specific radioimmunoassay using radiolabelled ethinyloestradiol. This method confirmed the results obtained with CIC, and the strong correlation between anti-EO ab and thrombosis (Fig. 16.1). Furthermore, in a previous study on 50 women with thrombosis and their controls anti-EO ab were found as the only risk factor in 44% of cases.

Antibody features: except for case 1 which was a monoclonal IgG λ, the anti-EO ab were always polyclonal IgGs. Fundamental analysis showed[13] that the Igs had binding activities for ethinyloestradiol, with a Ka ranging from $4.10^5 M^{-1}$ to $2.6.10^7 M^{-1}$, a valence of 2, which is consistent with the two binding sites of an Ig, and that the reactive part of the molecule was the Fab fragment.

The binding activity was maximal for ethinyloestradiol, but cross-reactivity with

195

17-beta-oestradiol, progesterone or other sex steroid hormones could be observed to a lesser degree.

It may be observed that the association constant of the antihormone antibodies is less strong than the affinity of hormone receptors, a finding that may explain why the presence of anti-EO ab does not inhibit contraception.

The antibodies were never found in women who had not used synthetic sex hormones. In users, they may be detected as early as the third week and in women with a low as well as a high oestrogen dosage. A follow-up of reactive women showed that the antibodies were regularly found throughout contraception and for years after discontinuation. The persistence of antibodies might account for the residual risk of thrombosis reported in ex-users.[15]

The role of the antibodies in the development of thrombosis is not clear. It may be pointed out that several reports on pathological findings in women on oral contraceptives emphasised the usual lack of atherosclerotic lesions and described vascular changes which may resemble the lesions of immunological or autoimmune disorders.[6, 19-22] The antibodies were shown to form circulating immune complexes which may damage the vascular endothelium, promote intimal modifications, enhance coagulation processes, and activate platelets, leading to thrombosis.

It is interesting that Rosenberg et al[23] found no relation between oestrogen use and MI in postmenopausal women treated with 'natural' equine oestrogen. In our experience, these oestrogens do not induce anti-EO ab.

SMOKING AND ORAL CONTRACEPTION

Cigarette smoking is a known risk factor in vascular disease in men as well as in women. Radford and Oliver[24] found that 47% of women with ischaemic heart disease under 45 years were smokers compared with 26% in the general population, and Kay et al[25] found that women on oral contraceptives smoked more than non-users.

The potentiating effect of cigarette smoking in the vascular risk of oral contraceptives was emphasised in many epidemiological studies,[12,15] especially in women with MI.[10,12,16,21,26,27] Previous studies[16] also showed that half the women with thrombosis and anti-EO ab were smokers and that, when compared with healthy users, smoking appeared to be an important factor only in women with antibodies. This seems to be confirmed in the present study, especially in MI (Table 16.6). The

Table 16.6 Respective role of antiethinyloestradiol antibodies and cigarette smoking.

Anti-EO ab: Cigarette smoking:		No No	No Yes	Yes No	Yes Yes
Cerebrovascular diseases (n cases)	19	2	1	8	8
Ischaemic heart diseases (n cases)	13	0	1	2	10
Venous thrombosis and/or pulmonary embolism (n cases)	17	1	1	9	6

suggestion might be advanced that the penetration of circulating immune complexes and/or antibodies through the vascular endothelium is facilitated by the increase in vascular permeability induced by nicotine.

CONCLUSION

Finally, except for smoking the risk factors for atherosclerosis, hypertension, diabetes, hypercholesterolaemia, do not seem to have an important role in the development of vascular lesions, which have usually not the characteristics of atheromatous lesions.[16,21] It must be realised, however, that they may play a part in older women on the pill and that, with time, the lesions induced by oral contraceptives may predispose to atherosclerosis. But they cannot predict the risk of cardiovascular side effects.

On the other hand, the determination of serum anti-EO ab among healthy users may define a group of women at risk.

The presence of the antibodies, which were shown to persist years after stopping the pill, might also account for the residual risk reported in several publications[12,27] (Table 16.7).

Table 16.7 Thrombosis in ex-users, residual risk.

Time from stopping (years)	No of cases	Anti-EO ab at the moment of thrombosis
<1	10	10
1-5	5	4
>5	4	3

SUMMARY

The risk of myocardial infarction (MI) is increased in women on oral contraceptives. The incidence of different risk factors predisposing to coronary heart disease was compared in 20 pill users with MI, 17 users with venous thrombosis and 19 users with an ischaemic cerebrovascular disease. Serum antibodies to synthetic sex hormones, which were shown to be correlated with thrombosis, were also determined in all cases.

Except for cigarette smoking, the prevalence of risk factors was very low. On the other hand, antibodies to synthetic sex hormones were the most common factor in women with MI as well as in thrombosis of other localisations. They were found in nearly 90% of cases.

It is concluded that the determination of risk factors cannot be predictive of the development of thrombosis in pill users, and that the detection of antihormone antibodies among healthy users may define a group of women at risk. The synergistic action of antibodies and cigarette smoking is also considered.

REFERENCES

[1] Report from the Boston Collaborative Drug Surveillance Programme. Oral contraceptives and venous thromboembolic disease, surgically confirmed gallbladder disease, and breast tumours. Lancet 1973; 1: 1399–1404.

[2] Collaborative Group for the Study of Stroke in Young Women. Oral contraception and increased risk of cerebral ischemia or thrombosis. N Engl J Med 1973; 288: 871–878.

[3] Royal College of General Practitioners' Oral Contraception Study. Mortality among oral-contraceptive users. Lancet 1977; 2: 727–31.

[4] Boyce J, Fawcett JW, Noall EWP. Coronary thrombosis and Conovid. Lancet 1963; 1: 111.

[5] Oliver MF. Oral contraceptives and myocardial infarction. Br Med J 1970; 2: 210–3.

[6] Weiss S. Myocardial infarction and oral contraceptives. N Engl J Med 1972; 286: 436–7.

[7] Benacerraf A, Veron P, Morin B, Castillo-Fenoy A, Chapuis A, Ziskind B. Infarctus du myocarde après contraceptifs oraux. Nouv Presse Med 1977; 6: 22–6.

[8] Bounhoure JP, Marco J, Fauvel JM et al. Contraceptifs oraux et infarctus du myocarde. Arch Mal Coeur 1977; 70: 765–71.

[9] Barrillon A, Delahaye JP, Grand A et al. Infarctus du myocarde et contraception orale. Arch Mal Coeur 1977; 70: 921–8.

[10] Mann JI, Vessey MP, Thorogood M, Doll R. Myocardial infarction in young women with special reference to oral contraceptive practice. Br Med J 1975; 2: 241–5.

[11] Mann JI, Inman WHW. Oral contraceptives and death from myocardial infarction. Br Med J 1975; 2: 245–8.

[12] Royal College of General Practitioners' Oral Contraception Study. Further analyses of mortality in oral contraceptive users. Lancet 1981;. 1: 541–6.

[13] Beaumont JL, Lemort N. Oral contraceptive, pulmonary artery thrombosis and anti-ethinyl-oestradiol monoclonal IgG. Clin Exp Immunol 1976; 24: 455–63.

[14] Beaumont V, Lemort N, Beaumont JL. Oral contraception, circulation immune complexes, antiethinylestradiol antibodies, and thrombosis. Am J Reprod Immunol 1982; 2: 8–12.

[15] Stadel BV. Oral contraceptives and cardiovascular disease. N Engl J Med 1981; 305: 672–7.

[16] Beaumont V, Lemort N, Beaumont JL. Evaluation of risk factors associated with vascular thrombosis in women on oral contraceptives. Possible role of anti-sex steroid hormone antibodies. Artery 1983; 11: 331–44.

[17] Beaumont V, Lemort N, Lorenzelli L, Mosser A, Beaumont JL. Hormones contraceptives, risque vasculaire et précipitabilité anormale des gammaglobulines sériques. Pathol Biol 1978; 26: 531–7.

[18] Beaumont V, Delplanque B, Lemort N, Beaumont JL. Blood changes in sex steroid hormone users. Circulating immune complexes induced by estrogens and progestogens and their relation to vascular thrombosis. Atherosclerosis 1982; 44: 343–53.

[19] Irey NS, Manion WC, Taylor HB. Vascular lesions in women taking oral contraceptives. Arch Pathol (Chicago) 1970; 89: 1–8.

[20] Dear HD, Jones WB. Myocardial infarction associated with the use of oral contraceptives. Ann Intern Med 1971; 74: 236–9.

[21] Bakouche P, Vedrenne C, Beaumont V, Chaouat D, Reignier A, Nick J. Thromboangéite à cellules géantes au cours d'une contraception orale. Etude anatomoclinique et immunologique. Rev Neurol (Paris) 1980; 136: 509–19.

[22] Engel H-J, Engel E, Lichtlen PR. Coronary atherosclerosis and myocardial infarction in young women—role of oral contraceptives. Eur Heart J 1983; 4: 1–18.

[23] Rosenberg L, Armstrong B, Phil D, Jick H. Myocardial infarction and estrogen therapy in post-menopausal women. N Engl J Med 1976; 294: 1256–9.

[24] Radford DJ, Oliver MF. Oral contraceptives and myocardial infarction. Br Med J 1973; 3: 428–30.

[25] Kay CR, Smith A, Richards B. Smoking habits of oral contraceptive users. Lancet 1969; 2: 1228–9.

[26] Jick H, Dinan B, Rothman KJ. Non-contraceptive estrogens and nonfatal myocardial infarction. J Am Med Assoc 1978; 239: 1407–8.

[27] Shapiro S, Slone D, Rosenberg L, Kaufman DW, Stolley PD, Miettinen OS. Oral-contraceptive use in relation to myocardial infarction. Lancet 1979; 1: 743–7.

[28] Slone D, Shapiro S, Kaufman DW, Rosenberg L, Miettinen OS, Stolley PD. Risk of myocardial infarction in relation to current and discontinued use of oral contraceptives. N Engl J Med 1981; 305: 420–4.

198

Discussion on Chapter 16

Oliver

Have you any evidence about false-positives?

Beaumont J.-L.

In our experience, with the radioimmunoassay (RIA) there are no false-positives regarding binding. When a positive result is found in a non-user after obtaining complete information it turns out that the woman has taken another synthetic sex hormone in the past. On the other hand, there are false-positive results with the immune complex detection method which is not specific for antihormone-antibody complexes. These 'false-positives' are more frequent in older age groups. Finally, one can say that the RIA is sensitive and specific and it must be kept in mind that positive results may reflect the use of a synthetic hormone which was stopped years before the test and may have been forgotten.

Sternby

In the first case you presented, I wonder if there were any other arterial lesions because it is uncommon to see coronary artery disease in a young girl? It indicates that she might have similar lesions elsewhere in the body.

Beaumont J.-L.

Yes, she had other localisation. In this case there was a diffuse arteritis.

Sternby

I think that some of the cases of thrombosis in pill-users may be due to either arteritis or to defects in the coagulation system. We have seen such cases where relatives have been found to have such defects. Something else is needed in addition to the pill. Arteritis might perhaps be initiated through immune complexes.

17. Sex differences in postinfarction prognosis and secondary risk factors

S. Johansson, G. Ulvenstam, A. Vedin and
C. Wilhelmsson

Similar postinfarction survival rates for women and men have been reported both during the first[1-3] and subsequent years of follow-up.[1,4,5] A poorer survival rate has also been proposed in female compared with male patients[6,7] but most studies mainly consider women aged over 50. Generally, the prognosis after myocardial infarction (MI) is less well documented for women than for men.

Several factors are associated with an unfavourable prognosis. It is well known that previous MI and factors associated with the severity of the myocardial damage all contribute to a poor prognosis. Previous work mainly in men has also shown that the major risk factors, tobacco smoking,[8,9] hypertension[10] and hypercholesterolaemia,[11] remain as risk factors for recurrent events.

This study will focus on the long-term prognosis in women aged under 65 at the time of first infarction. Comparisons are made with the prognosis in men from the same population. The importance of hypertension, total serum cholesterol, angina pectoris and diabetes mellitus for the long-term prognosis were analysed. Mortality and non-fatal reinfarctions are the chief prognostic endpoints.

MATERIAL AND METHODS

Registration of all cases of MI occurring in the population of Göteborg (450 000) has been in operation since January 1968.[12] All patients were systematically followed up at a special post-MI clinic.[13] The present study consisted of women and men discharged from hospital after a first MI between 1 January 1968 and 31 December 1977. During the follow-up, examinations and interviews took place at clinically determined intervals and always 1, 3, 12, 24, 60 and 120 months after the MI. For all interviews and physical examinations identical questionnaires were used by the same group of investigators. Patients were treated according to uniform rules established by means of regular staff meetings.

Among secondary preventive measures, antismoking information, treatment of hypertension and prophylactic beta-blockade after the MI in the annual cohorts 1975–77 were emphasised. Patients with cholesterol levels above 7.8 mmol/l 3 months after MI were given general dietary advice. Drug treatment was given to not more than 8% of the patients in the highest cholesterol quintile. Coronary bypass surgery was performed in not more than 3% of any annual cohort.

Deaths and non-fatal reinfarctions were verified by the MI register through continuous checking of all death certificates and hospital records of all patients admitted with symptoms suggestive of MI. At the end of the follow-up period the survival status of all patients was known. The patients were followed to December 1979.

Hypertension was considered to be present if the patient had previously been informed by a physician that the blood pressure was raised; or the blood pressure measured 3 months after MI was diastolic>105 and/or systolic>160 mm Hg or if the patient received treatment for hypertension 3 months after the MI. Angina pectoris was recorded if the patient had experienced chest pain on physical effort for longer than 1 month before MI. Diabetes before MI was recorded if the patient had previously been diagnosed by a physician as suffering from diabetes. Definitions of other clinical variables have been published previously.[12,13] Total serum cholesterol was determined after 12 hours' fasting 3 months after MI.[14]

Fisher's permutation test was used to test differences in continuous and binary variables. For binary variables, this test is equivalent to Fisher's test in a fourfold table.[15] To make use of all information the Kaplan-Meier estimate was used to produce survival curves.[16] The log rank procedure was used to test differences between survival curves.[17]

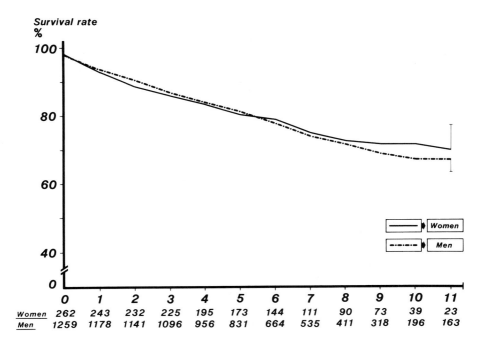

Fig. 17.1 Survival curves for women and men with a first myocardial infarction. The numbers below the time axis denote the number of patients at the beginning of each interval.

RESULTS

During the 10 year period 1968–77 262 women (mean age 54.4±6.1) and 1259 men (mean age 52.9±6.2) were discharged from hospital after a first MI (Table 17.1). During the maximal possible observation period of 12 years, 65 women and 327 men died. 80% of the deaths were attributable to cardiovascular diseases.

Table 17.1 Numbers of women and men with a first non-fatal myocardial infarction 1968–77.

Age (years)	Women n	Women %	Men n	Men %
-44	20	7.7	122	9.7
45–49	28	10.7	196	15.6
50–54	70	26.7	374	29.7
55–59	91	34.7	421	33.4
60–64	53	20.2	146	11.6
Total	262	100	1259	100

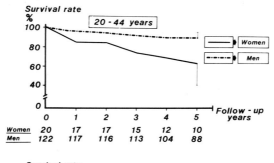

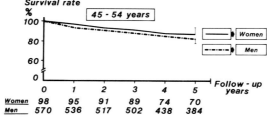

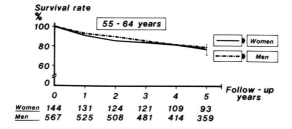

Fig. 17.2 Survival curves for women and men with a first myocardial infarction within three different age groups.

The cumulative survival rate during follow-up was similar in women and men (Fig. 17.1). The survival rate decreased with advancing age in men (p < 0.01; Fig. 17.2), but women aged under 45 were associated with the lowest survival rate. For patients aged under 45 the cumulative 5 year survival rate was lower in women (64%) than in men (91%; p < 0.01). The survival rate was similar in older patients.

During the follow-up period, 63 women and 308 men suffered a non-fatal reinfarction. The cumulative 5 year non-fatal recurrence rate was similar in the two sexes, being 21% in women and 24% in men (Fig. 17.3). The recurrence rate was not related to age.

A history of hypertension was more common in women (40%) than in men (23%; p < 0.001). The female patients also had a higher mean systolic blood pressure (152±24 mm Hg) 3 months after infarction than the male patients (144±22 mm Hg; p<0.001). In all, 154 women (59%) and 475 men (38%) had hypertension.

The hypertensive women were older (mean age 55.0±6.0) than those without hypertension (53.4±6.3; p<0.05). No difference was found in the primary risk factors—tobacco smoking and total serum cholesterol—or in the clinical characteristics—congestive heart failure or maximal enzyme release—in the two groups studied.

Survival curves in relation to hypertension are shown in Figure 17.4. The cumulative survival rate 5 years after MI was 79% in hypertensive women compared with 83% in those without hypertension (p=0.193). The corresponding 5 year survival rate for men with hypertension was 77% and for those without hypertension 84% (p=0.004). The cumulative reinfarction rate after 5 years was 26% in hypertensive women and 20% in nonhypertensives (p=0.098; Fig. 17.5). The 5 year

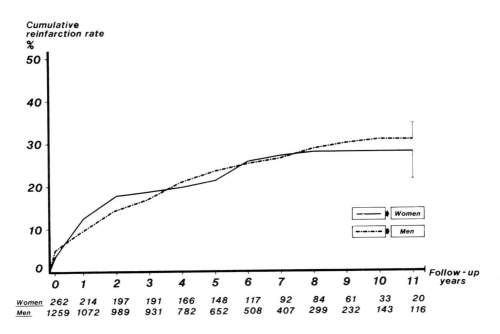

Fig. 17.3 Cumulative reinfarction rates for women and men with a first myocardial infarction.

recurrence rate was 30% for men with hypertension and 19% for those without hypertension (p < 0.001).

Mean values of serum cholesterol 3 months after infarction were higher in the female (7.4±1.7 mmol/l; p < 0.001). The difference was confined to patients aged 50 years and over.

The female patients were divided into serum cholesterol tertile groups according to the 3 month postinfarction serum cholesterol value. Mean serum cholesterol in the lowest tertile was 5.9 mmol/l and in the highest tertile 9.1 mmol/l. No

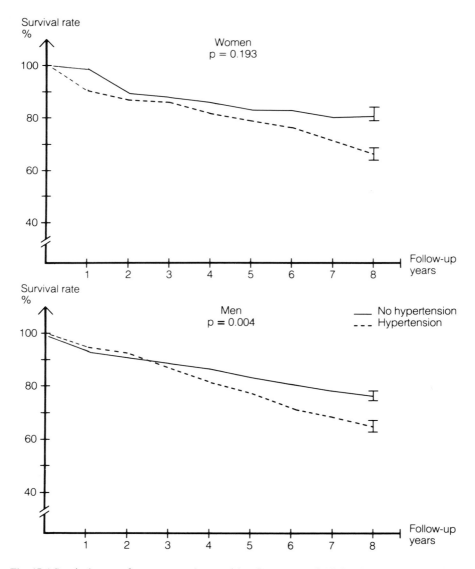

Fig. 17.4 Survival curves for women and men with a first myocardial infarction in relation to hypertension.

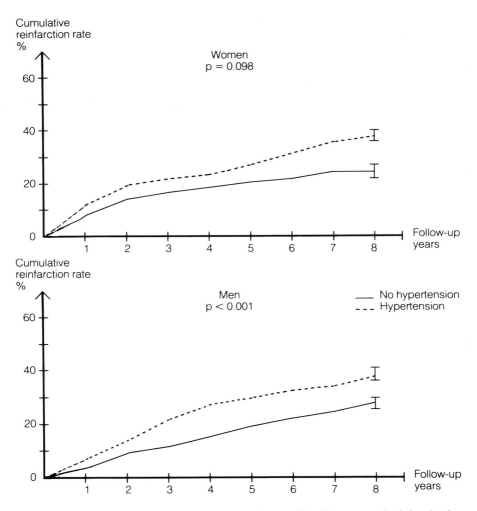

Fig. 17.5 Cumulative reinfarction rates for women and men with a first myocardial infarction in relation to hypertension.

association was found between tobacco consumption, hypertension, congestive heart failure or maximal enzyme release and serum cholesterol tertiles in women. The 5 year cumulative survival rate was 84%, 78% and 79%, respectively, in the lowest, intermediate, and highest cholesterol tertile groups (Fig. 17.6). Serum cholesterol was not related to the recurrence rate in women (Fig. 17.7). No sex difference was observed in either survival or recurrence rate in relation to cholesterol tertiles.

Angina pectoris before infarction was as common in women as in men. At the time of infarction 100 women (39%) and 368 men (31%) had angina pectoris. The female patients with angina were somewhat older (mean age 55.2±5.5) than those without (54.0±6.3; p < 0.01). No significant differences were found with regard to hypertension, total serum cholesterol, congestive heart failure or maximal enzyme release but women with angina were less often smokers (52%) than those without (70%; p < 0.01).

The survival rate in women was not associated with angina pectoris (Fig. 17.8). The 5 year cumulative survival rate in men was 74% for those with angina pectoris and 86% for those without (p < 0.001). The recurrence rate after 5 years in women

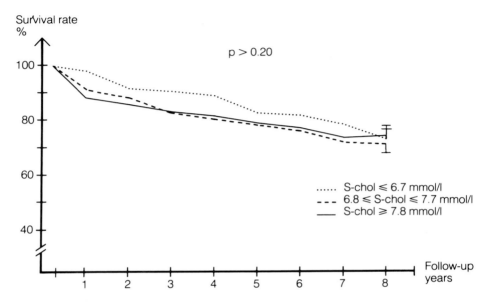

Fig. 17.6 Survival curves for women with a first myocardial infarction in relation to serum cholesterol.

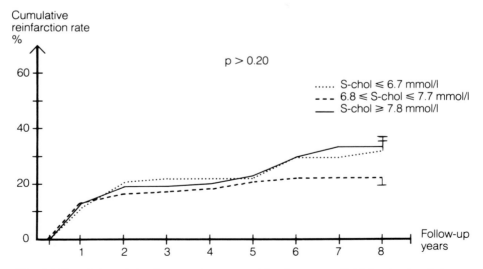

Fig. 17.7 Cumulative reinfarction rates for women with a first myocardial infarction in relation to serum cholesterol.

206

with angina pectoris was 23% compared with 33% in those without angina (p=0.005; Fig. 17.9). The corresponding recurrence rate in men with angina pectoris was 25% as compared with 35% in those without angina (p < 0.001).

At the time of infarction 20 women (8%) and 73 men (6%) had diabetes (p > 0.20). Below age 45 diabetes was more common in women (5/20; 25%) compared with men (6/122; 5%).

The female diabetics were younger at the time of infarction (51.3±8.5) than non-diabetics (54.6±5.8; p<0.05). The primary risk factors—tobacco smoking,

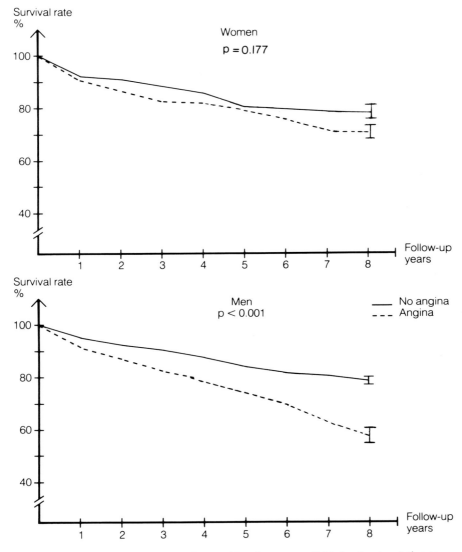

Fig. 17.8 Survival curves for women and men with a first myocardial infarction in relation to angina pectoris.

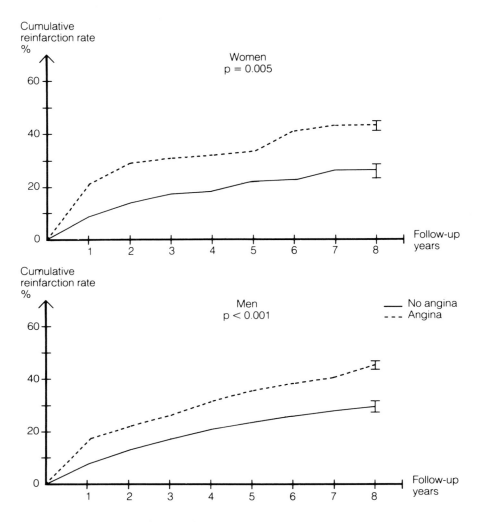

Fig. 17.9 Cumulative reinfarction rates for women and men with a first myocardial infarction in relation to angina pectoris.

hypertension and serum cholesterol—differed between the groups, tobacco smoking being more common among non-diabetic women (p<0.001) and hypertension more common among diabetic women (p < 0.1). No difference was found in clinical characteristics such as congestive heart failure or maximal enzyme release.

Survival curves in relation to diabetes are shown in Figure 17.10. The cumulative survival rate 5 years after infarction was 65% for diabetic women and 82% for those without diabetes (p=0.004). Diabetes was also associated with a lower survival rate in men. The 5 year recurrence rate in women with diabetes was 38% compared with 26% in those without diabetes (p > 0.20; Fig. 17.11). The corresponding 5 year recurrence rate was 27% in diabetic men compared with 47% in those without diabetes (p=0.002).

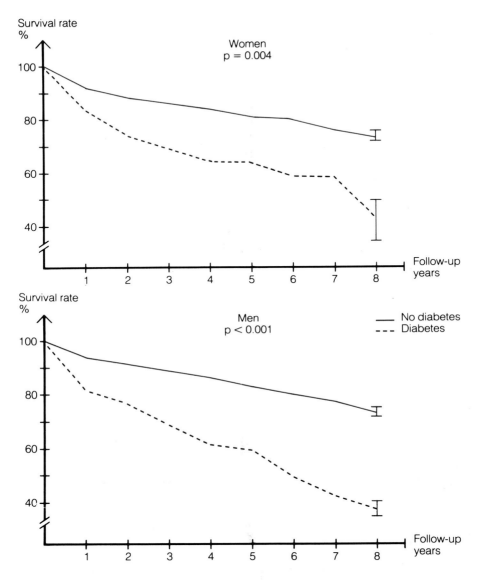

Fig. 17.10 Survival curves for women and men with a first myocardial infarction in relation to diabetes.

DISCUSSION

The patients in the present study were representative of the middle-aged population in Göteborg. More than 90% of all MI cases were entered on the MI register.[12] The methods for registration and follow-up were unchanged.[12,13] The present study was confined to patients who survived an MI, and data concerning deaths before or during hospital stay were not available.

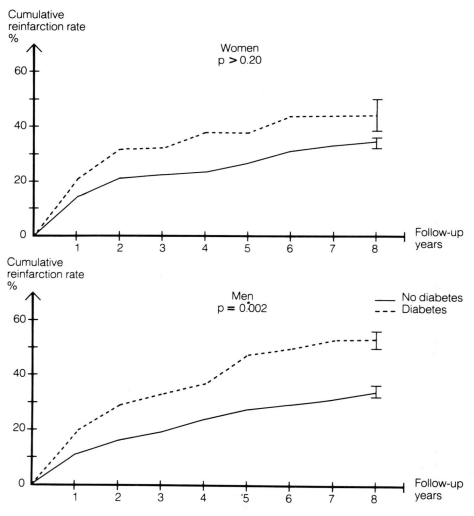

Fig. 17.11 Cumulative reinfarction rates for women and men with a first myocardial infarction in relation to diabetes.

A 5 year postinfarction survival of about 80% in women previously reported [1,4,18] confirms the present rates for women aged over 45. A similar long-term survival in women and men aged over 45 is also in accordance with most previous studies. [1,4] A lower postinfarction survival in women aged under 45 has been suggested in one previous study. [19]

The low number of young female patients in this study necessitates caution in the interpretation of the results. Sex differences in the risk factor load before infarction, with an overrepresentation of hypertension and diabetes in women compared with men, [20] may influence the long-term prognosis. Despite a 10 year sampling period the low incidence of MI among young women does not permit comparisons of patients with a similar risk factor load.

210

The importance of serum cholesterol,[11] diabetes mellitus,[21] angina pectoris and hypertension[10] for the prognosis after infarction has been studied in more detail in the male patients in this infarction series. Because of the higher number of male patients multivariate statistics were possible. The worse prognosis among male patients in relation to diabetes, total serum cholesterol, hypertension and angina pectoris remained when adjustments were made for possible confounding factors in preinfarction characteristics and factors of secondary prognostic importance.

In defining hypertension, the hypertensive status after as well as before MI was used as a number of patients with undetected hypertension or with hypertension of recent onset would otherwise have been missed. Some misclassification could still be possible as the MI itself decreases the blood pressure and this implies that the prognostic differences between the studied groups may decrease. The role of hypertension in the prognosis among women has been debated.[1] In the HIP study[1] hypertension was not related to the long-term mortality in women but had an unfavourable influence on the prognosis in men. The survival rate was similar in women and men with hypertension in this study although possibly because of small numbers the difference between women with and without hypertension did not reach statistical significance. Hypertension in women seemed to be a more predisposing factor for reinfarctions rather than for death.

High levels of serum cholesterol have been associated with a poor prognosis in women[1] which was not observed in this study. Among men, however, an association between cholesterol levels and the long-term mortality was observed only in those aged under 50 at the time of first infarction.[11]

SUMMARY

Young women aged under 45 seemed to have a poorer prognosis than men of similar ages. In part this can be due to there being comparatively more diabetic women than men in this age group. The similar occurrence of non-fatal reinfarctions and deaths during follow-up in patients aged over 45 indicates that once women have suffered a myocardial infarction (MI) they are exposed to at least as high a risk as men. The presence of diabetes, and probably hypertension, is of importance for recurrent fatal events after infarction. The relatively high mortality during follow-up in relation to angina pectoris in men was not seen in the female patients. This factor, however, may be of some importance in predicting non-fatal events in women.

REFERENCES

[1]Weinblatt E, Shapiro S, Frank CW. Prognosis of women with newly diagnosed coronary heart disease—a comparison with course of disease among men. Am J Publ Health 1973; 63: 577–93.
[2]World Health Organization. Myocardial infarction community registers. Public Health in Europe No 5. Copenhagen: WHO, 1976.
[3]Peter T, Harper R, Luxton M, Penington C, Sloman JG. Acute myocardial infarction in women. The influence of age on complications and mortality. Med J Aust 1978; 1: 189–91.
[4]Kannel WB, Sorlie P, McNamara PM. Prognosis after initial myocardial infarction: the Framingham study. Am J Cardiol 1979; 44: 53–9.
[5]Henning R, Wedel H. The long-term prognosis after myocardial infarction: a five year follow-up study. Eur Heart J 1981; 2: 65–74.

[6]Juergens JL, Edwards JE, Achor RWP, Burchell HB. Prognosis of patients surviving first clinically diagnosed myocardial infarction. Arch Intern Med 1960; 105: 444–50.

[7]Thygesen K, Dalsgaard P, Lyager Nielsen B. Prognosis after first myocardial infarction. Acta Med Scand 1974; 195: 253–9.

[8]Aberg A, Bergstrand R, Johansson S et al. Cessation of smoking after myocardial infarction. Effects on mortality after 10 years. Br Heart J 1983; 49: 416–22.

[9]Johansson S, Bergstrand R, Pennert K et al. Cessation of smoking after myocardial infarction in women. Effects on mortality and reinfarctions. Am J Epidemiol 1985; 121: 823–31.

[10]Ulvenstam G, Aberg A, Bergstrand R et al. Prognostic importance of hypertension and chronic angina pectoris in survivors of myocardial infarction. Submitted.

[11]Ulvenstam G, Bergstrand R, Johansson S et al. Prognostic importance of cholesterol levels after myocardial infarction. Prev Med 1984; 13: 355–66.

[12]Elmfeldt D, Wilhelmsen L, Tibblin G, Vedin JA, Wilhelmsson C-E, Bengtsson C. Registration of myocardial infarction in the city of Göteborg, Sweden. A community study. J Chronic Dis 1975; 28: 173–86.

[13]Elmfeldt D, Wilhelmsen L, Tibblin G, Vedin A, Wilhelmsson C-E, Bengtsson C. A postmyocardial infarction clinic in Göteborg, Sweden. A follow-up of MI patients in a specialized out-patient clinic. Acta Med Scand 1975; 197–502.

[14]Cramér K, Isaksson B. An evaluation of the Theorell method for the determination of total serum cholesterol. Scand J Clin Lab Invest 1959; 11: 213–6.

[15]Bradley JV. Distribution-free statistical tests. Englewood Cliffs, New Jersey: Prentice-Hall, 1968: 68–86.

[16]Kaplan EL, Meier P. Nonparametric estimation from incomplete observations. J Am Stat Assoc 1958; 53: 457–81.

[17]Kalbfleisch JD, Prentice RL. The statistical analysis of failure time data. New York, Chichester, Brisbane, Toronto: John Wiley and Sons, 1980.

[18]Pohjola S, Siltanen P, Romo M. Five-year survival of 728 patients after myocardial infarction. Br Heart J 1980; 43: 176–83.

[19]Oliver MF. Clinical characteristics and prognosis of angina and myocardial infarction in young women. In: Oliver MF, ed. Coronary heart disease in young women. Edinburgh, London, New York: Churchill Livingstone, 1978: 221–32.

[20]Johansson S, Bergstrand R, Ulvenstam G et al. Sex differences in preinfarction characteristics and long-term survival among patients with myocardial infarction. Am J Epidemiol 1984; 119: 610–23.

[21]Ulvenstam G, Aberg A, Bergstrand R et al. Long-term prognosis after myocardial infarction in men with diabetes. Diabetes 1985; 34: 787–92.

Discussion on chapter 17

Bengtsson
What were the reasons for death in those young women?

Johansson
Cardiovascular deaths in 80%.

Epstein
Did I understand correctly that in this youngest age group where women had a worse survival rate than men it would have been more similar if it were not for diabetes? Of course the numbers are small.

Johansson
It could be, yes.

Haynes
Did you attempt to use multivariate analysis such as Cox regression to determine which of these risk factors were most important in predicting survival among the youngest women?

Johansson
We cannot do that because of the small number.

Haynes
Were any surgical procedures conducted among the women, in hospital and after their myocardial infarction? There has been some evidence in the United States that women who go through coronary bypass surgery may not fare as well as men, or that women who have a balloon catheterisation actually have 30% higher mortality after the procedure than men. An analysis of the medical care procedures used for the younger women might be instructive.

Johansson
No woman in the youngest age group underwent coronary bypass surgery and it is uncommon in this material. None underwent haemodynamic monitoring.

Vedin
I think it is important for our transatlantic visitors to realise that in this series no woman underwent any surgical procedure during the initial hospital phase and very few women, less than 5% in the entire series, during the 10 years of follow-up.

Wilhelmsson
The picture is changing but the latest follow-up here was at the end of 1979 so we have to note these figures.

Wynn
Were any of the younger women taking the pill when they had their myocardial infarction?

Johansson

No, none, but the material was recruited between 1968 and 1977 and none of the women were taking the pill.

Wilhelmsson

We also have other Swedish series on female myocardial infarction patients below 45 years of age in which around 30% of the female patients are taking the pill.

Wynn

What would be quite interesting, I think, would be to see what the survival rate and reinfarction rate is in these women if they stop taking the pill.

Wilhelmsson

The only thing I can say is that the survival rate after 2 years of follow-up in these young women is enormously good, almost 100%.

Haynes

I think the presenter should be congratulated in her excellent data in this relatively unexplored area. I have one additional question: do you have any details about the social support that these women received after myocardial infarction? There has been some preliminary evidence suggesting that if a woman has a myocardial infarction she does not receive the same social support as a man who has had a myocardial infarction.

Johansson

We don't have that yet for this group of patients, but we have a study in progress that is looking at that.

18. What is the difference between women and men? (Summary of closing comments)

M.F. Oliver

This is an important question so far as coronary heart disease (CHD) is concerned, even in these days of unisex. Why is the incidence lower? There are at least four possible explanations:
— a lower prevalence of risk factors in women than in men
— a better tolerance of risk factors when they are present
— hormonal and metabolic differences which give relative protection
— differences in clinical presentation
All of these are bound to influence the incidence.

PREVALENCE OF RISK FACTORS

Cigarette smoking is associated with lower CHD rates in women than in men but, interestingly, the gradient of difference in CHD from non-smokers to heavy smokers is not actually different between women and men.[1]

For blood pressure, again using the Framingham data,[1] there is quite an appreciable difference between men and women in the relationship of systolic and diastolic blood pressure to CHD. The lower prevalence of CHD in those with raised blood pressure does not, however, apply to stroke, for there is no such disparity between the sexes.

The Lipid Research Clinics[2] have provided useful data concerning the changes in plasma cholesterol with age. There are lower levels of cholesterol and lower levels of low-density lipoproteins (LDL) in adult women than in men, although the Framingham study did not show any difference in the significance of the positive regression of events on LDL between men and women. There are also higher high-density lipoprotein (HDL) concentrations in women. There is a negative relationship of considerable strength between LDL and stroke for women but not for men. The prevalence of atherogenic lipoprotein factors would appear to be different and more favourable for women.

From a personal survey[3] of 145 women under the age of 45, of whom 81 had had infarction and 64 had angina with positive ECG, there was more relationship between cigarette smoking and infarction than in angina, although the prevalences of raised cholesterol and diastolic pressure were similar. Other risk factors, such as a premature menopause and oral contraception, were more important in those with infarction than in those presenting with angina.

Hence, there is less smoking, lower blood pressure levels and a lower LDL/HDL ratio in adult women than in men and therefore a lower prevalence of risk factors. This is also true of obesity. Might there also be other major sex differences in, for example, LDL-receptor formation or in platelet-fibrin interaction?

ARE RISK FACTORS BETTER TOLERATED BY WOMEN?

One answer to the difference in CHD between men and women may be genetic, with genetic protection being greater in women. Women with severe polymorphic hypercholesterolaemia tolerate it better and live appreciably longer than men with the same disorder. Whether the clinical expression of CHD in men with FH is more dependent on the presence of other risk factors is not clear, although these are more prevalent in men.

Data from coronary arteriography, dependent on selection factors as it is, suggest a lower occurrence of obstructive disease for a given level of serum cholesterol in women. This also suggests that women may tolerate raised cholesterol better than men. At 7.8 mmol/l there is about half the amount of occlusion in women than there is in men. This applies also to all groups and all degrees of occlusion.

PROTECTION OF HORMONAL FACTORS

It is not new to suggest that hormonal factors may be protecting women from CHD, but they are seldom described. In 1953 we identified cyclical changes in plasma cholesterol and ester cholesterol during the menstrual cycle.[4] We measured these lipids and also phospholipids every day over a period of 5 weeks in 12 healthy women. Ovulation was identified by the waking morning temperature rise. Assembling the lipid changes around that temperature rise, we were able to show a striking and rather rapid fall in total cholesterol and of ester cholesterol but no change in free cholesterol at the time of ovulation. This study has not been repeated in order to examine changes in LDL and HDL. In terms of incidence of CHD, we should note that there are lower levels of plasma lipids, and cyclical changes, in women during the 30–40 years of their lives than in men.

These changes can be related to maintained physiological ovarian function. Compared with unilateral ovariectomy, bilateral ovariectomy carried out under the age of 35 is associated in later years with a higher incidence of CHD.[5] The CHD rate was 25% by the age of 50 compared with 3% in those with unilateral ovariectomy. Similarly, a spontaneous premature menopause[6] or secondary amenorrhoea has also been associated with an excess of CHD occurring about 10 years after the cessation of menstruation.

Another point: we assume that the rise in plasma cholesterol during pregnancy[7] is harmless and, evolutionarily, it should be true. But the rise is considerable—on average about 60%—and in some women serum cholesterol may rise into the top decile of its distribution in the normal population. The differences in plasma lipids between men and women are summarised in Figure 18.1.

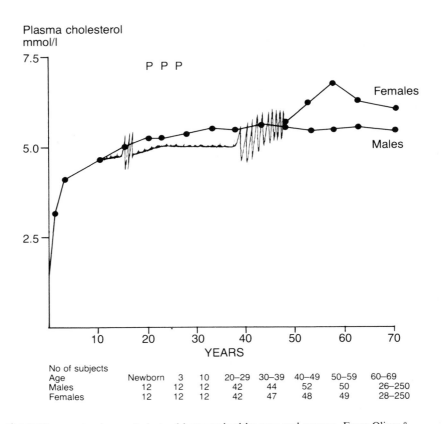

Fig. 18.1 Differences in plasma cholesterol between healthy men and women. From Oliver.[9]

In 500 consecutive patients with myocardial infarction who were compared with 500 controls—also a consecutive group and of the same age—there were more unmarried people among those with CHD. Among the unmarried women, more in the coronary group had had four or more pregnancies than those in the control group. Winkelstein et al[8] too found a higher parity rate, and also more abortions in women with CHD. We should not therefore totally dismiss the possibility that multiparity may have an adverse influence, although men with CHD also have more children!

DIFFERENCES IN CLINICAL PRESENTATION

Another explanation as to why CHD incidence is lower in women is that there may be differences in presentation. Of those who developed CHD in the Framingham study,[9] a majority of women (65%) and a minority of men (37%) presented with angina.

There are striking differences in the international trends in CHD mortality between the sexes,[10] with those for women falling in most WHO countries since 1950 and those for men showing no consistent pattern.

Recent trends in case-fatality figures show no differences between the sexes. The Minnesota Heart Study showed that the same reduction is taking place, presumably as a result of the same improvement in services for both men and women. The male/female ratio for CHD is higher for sudden cardiac death in younger age groups but we do not know whether there is a difference by sex in sudden cardiac death or the likelihood of getting ventricular fibrillation compared with infarction.

Dr Wilhelmsson suggested that the prognosis is different and worse in women. In my small study I am able to confirm this. While the prognosis in women under the age of 45 with angina and women under the age of 45 with infarction is similar, both are worse than those for men under 40 (published by Gertler et al[11] some years ago).

Are there sex differences in terms of haemostatic factors or the risk of thrombosis? That seems to be unanswerable because we cannot measure haemostatic factors with any great accuracy. Only now have we got emergent information about prospective studies[12] concerning the prediction of thrombosis, and today there is little fresh data available although thrombosis may be the commonest trigger for acute heart attack. Is it less common in women?

ARE OESTROGENS SAFE?

It is incumbent on the medical community to find out what will be the long-term effect of oral contraceptives—and, for that matter, of oestrogen replacement therapy—and to find it out soon.[13] We will be criticised harshly in the year 2000 for advising the use of oral contraceptives or oestrogen replacement therapy—particularly oral contraceptives—for social reasons without monitoring what might be happening. There is already evidence of adverse effects in the community of another social convenience pill, namely tranquillisers, and I think it is high time that a more precise and careful survey on the safety of oestrogens was conducted in several countries. It is difficult to establish a sound database. No country has got information—other than the prescription rates—to permit identification of a given woman, aged 25, and follow her through for 24 or 30 years knowing she is taking the same preparation and knowing that she is taking it regularly.

CHD PREVENTION IN WOMEN

How relevant is risk factor control in women? We have always assumed until now, tacitly I think, that what we advise for men should also be advised for women but, if the risk factor prevalence in women is indeed lower and if women tolerate the risk factors better, does it follow that the same measures should apply to women as to men? No major intervention trials have been conducted in women and the results of trials in men of different forms of intervention are fairly disappointing. Does it follow that we should ask women throughout the world to modify their lifestyle in the same way as we should ask men? If men are to alter their diet, perhaps the whole family should change; this is a pragmatic approach. But purely from a scientific point of view, there are not strong enough grounds for altering lifestyle in women.

Nevertheless, it would be a narrow scientific view not to recommend in unequivocal terms that women should reduce their consumption of cigarettes. No physician or epidemiologist should view the steady increase in cigarette smoking over the last 20 years, particularly by young women, with anything but alarm and concern.

REFERENCES

[1]Dawber TR. The Framingham Study. Cambridge, Mass: Howard University Press, 1980.

[2]Davis CE, Gordon D, LaRosa J, Wood PDS, Halperin M. Correlations of plasma high-density lipoprotein cholesterol levels with other plasma lipid and lipoprotein concentrations. The Lipid Research Clinics Program Prevalence Study. Circulation 1980; 5: 24–30.

[3]Oliver MF, Boyd GS. Endocrine aspects of coronary sclerosis. Lancet 1956; 2: 1273–6.

[4]Oliver MF, Boyd GS. Changes in the plasma lipids during menstrual cycle. Clin Sci 1952; 12: 217–22.

[5]Oliver MF, Boyd GS. Effect of bilateral ovariectomy on coronary-artery disease and serum-lipid levels. Lancet 1959; 2: 690–4.

[6]Sznajderman M, Oliver MF. Spontaneous premature menopause, ischaemic heart-disease, and serum-lipids. Lancet 1963; 1: 962–5.

[7]Oliver MF, Boyd GS. Plasma lipid and serum lipoprotein patterns during pregnancy and puerperium. Clin Sci 1955; 14: 15–23.

[8]Winkelstein W Jr, Stenchever MA, Lilienfeld AM. Occurrence of pregnancy, abortion, and artificial menopause among women with coronary artery disease: a preliminary study. J Chronic Dis 1958; 7: 273–86.

[9]Kannel WB, Feinleib M. Natural history of angina pectoris in the Framingham study. Am J Cardiol 1972; 29: 154–86.

[10]Thom I, Epstein FH, Feldman JJ, Leaverton PE. Trends in total mortality and mortality from heart disease in 26 countries 1950–78. Int J Epidemiol 1985.

[11]Gertler MM, White PD, Simon R, Gottsch LG. Long-term follow-up study of young coronary patients. Am J Med Sci 1964; 247: 145–55.

[12]Meade TW. Clotting factors and ischaemic heart disease—the epidemiological evidence. In Meade TW, ed Anticoagulants and myocardial infarction. John Wiley & Sons, London, p 91–112.

[13]Oliver MF. Oral contraceptives and coronary heart disease. In Julian DG, Wenger NK, eds Cardiac problems of the adolescent and young adult. Butterworth, London 197–212.

219

Discussion on chapter 18

Wilhelmsson
I wonder if you are right when you pose the question why the incidence is lower in women. Perhaps the question will change to why the incidence is higher in men. Do you think that is the same thing?

Oliver
It is an equally relevant question and isn't necessarily the same thing.

Sternby
When you talked about the higher tolerance in women it reminded me of an interesting finding. If you look at coronary heart disease deaths in various populations and you look at the coronary atherosclerosis, you find different levels according to the general level in the populations. For instance, if you look at the coronary victims in Norway they have a much higher level of atherosclerosis than they have in South America. I do not know of any similar studies regarding men and women. I have no explanation but it seems that the rate of coronary heart disease is related to the general level of atherosclerosis. Of course, it is well known that if you take men dying of myocardial infarction, let us say before 50, they have the same amount of atherosclerosis as men dying of myocardial infarction at the age of 80. There seems to be a level above which you are very prone to develop atherosclerosis. I think that has implications for the general health of the population because if you can lower the level of atherosclerosis you will automatically lower the frequency of coronary heart disease.

Haynes
I would like to congratulate you, Dr Oliver, on your excellent summary. One important point you raised is the issue of the effects of pregnancy and number of children on myocardial infarction. As a point of clarification, when you looked at unmarried women in your study, did the unmarried women include the separated, divorced and widowed? That might explain why you had a higher rate of disease in that particular group. If you had looked at the single women by themselves you might not have found excess risks.

Oliver
In that series the unmarried women were single, never married, and never divorced. They were spinsters.

Haynes
Bengtsson and co-workers published a Swedish study of women with myocardial infarction and showed that women with myocardial infarction were significantly more likely to have had four or more children. I think it is important to look at what occurs during pregnancy. If it increases cholesterol, perhaps platelet-aggregation or some other biological mechanism causes an increased atherogenic profile for some women.

Oliver

I am rather confused about this. One report on women who had been killed accidentally when they were in advanced pregnancy showed they had got a lot of lipid lesions, a lot of fatty streaks in the aorta and in the coronary arteries. The popular view is that fatty streaks are not relevant in terms of formation of fibrous lesions and therefore we perhaps could dismiss this, but I doubt it. Because after we did that series of trials we looked rather more closely and more carefully at some women than others. I was interested in what happens to cholesterol and low-density lipoproteins (LDL) when we were able to measure LDL in women during pregnancy. These levels go enormously high. You frequently get levels of about 8–9 mmol/l about the 7th or 8th month. HDL does not go up proportionately with LDL.

Haynes

As you noted, the technology for measuring platelet-aggregation, fibrinogen, and the various clotting factors is still not advanced. About 5 years ago the National Heart, Lung, and Blood Institute held a symposium, edited by Dr McMillan and others, where they commented on the technology of platelet function tests and on platelet functioning and platelet factors. At that time, no sex differences were found in platelet-aggregation. It could have been a methodological difference in measuring platelets. Perhaps platelets cling to the container or to the syringe more when the blood is drawn. So far the evidence has not been too promising in that field.

Index